## Praise for Bradie S. Crandall

"*The Living Machine* is a calculated look at the human body as a mechanical object and how a plant-based diet might be the ideal fuel for power and performance as well as health. Finally, a book that explains in great detail how an increasing number of athletes have been able to thrive on a vegan diet, without exaggeration or pseudoscience. This is the manual for plant-based performance I wish I'd had when I started."

-**Nick Squires**, 2019 International Powerlifting League World Champion

"The poster dude of powerful veganism…[Bradie is] competing in a strength sport amongst non-vegans and showing us all how it's done."

-**Karina Inkster**, fitness and nutrition coach, author, and host of the No Bullsh!t Vegan podcast

"[Bradie] consumes no animal products and yet he has extraordinary levels of muscle mass and performs darn well in the gym. Could it be that protein exists outside of meat? Could it be that soy doesn't "feminize" your hormone profile? Could there even be BENEFITS to going vegan?"

-**Nick English**, *BarBend News*

"The book is impressive…I hope people are willing to learn and give it [plant-based diets] a shot"

-**Ryan Woods**, comedian and host of the Into The Woods podcast

# The Living Machine

## Engineering Strength with a Plant-Based Diet

Bradie S. Crandall

**Disclaimer:**

The advice provided in the following text is based upon the dietary perspective and interpretations of a single individual. The advice is not intended to treat any specific medical condition or illness. Anything that could be interpreted as advice in this book is for informational purposes only. The material presented should not be used as a substitute nor replacement for professional medical advice. A physician or other healthcare professional should always be consulted prior to beginning a new diet or fitness program.

First printed in the United States of America

by CreateSpace, July 2020

Copyright © 2020 Bradie S. Crandall

Thank you for purchasing an authorized copy of this book.

No part of this book may be reproduced in any form or by any means without the prior consent of the publisher, except for brief quotes used in reviews.

ISBN: 9798654269256

Designed by Bradie S. Crandall

Cover Art by JohnLee Barnett

Editing by Jacob Chester

**"Our body is a machine for living. It is organized for that, it is its nature."**

-Leo Tolstoy

*This book is dedicated to all living beings.*

# Contents

| | |
|---|---|
| Acknowledgements............................................ | (1) |
| A Note to Readers............................................. | (2) |
| Introduction.................................................... | (6) |
| 1. The Experiment........................................... | (9) |
| 2. The Next Generation of Athletes..................... | (14) |
| 3. The Plant-Based Edge.................................. | (17) |
|     Increased Micronutrient Intake................... | (18) |
|     Decreased Consumption of Junk Food.......... | (22) |
|     Improved Microbiome............................. | (24) |
|     Faster Recovery.................................... | (26) |
|     Enhanced Blood Flow............................. | (29) |
|     The Chip on the Shoulder Effect................. | (33) |
| 4. Protein..................................................... | (35) |
|     How Much Do I Need?............................ | (36) |
|     Amino Acids....................................... | (38) |
|     The Truth About Soy.............................. | (39) |
|     Plant-Based Protein Sources..................... | (43) |
|     Protein Powder.................................... | (48) |
| 5. Carbs vs. Fat............................................ | (52) |
| 6. Reframing Diet ......................................... | (56) |
| 7. Supplementation........................................ | (60) |
|     Essential............................................ | (61) |
|     Recommended..................................... | (64) |
|     Optional............................................. | (69) |
| 8. Plant-based Strength Masters......................... | (77) |
|     Patrik Baboumian.................................. | (78) |
|     Nimai Delgado..................................... | (79) |
|     Nick Squires....................................... | (80) |
|     Kendrick Farris.................................... | (83) |
|     Honorable Mentions............................... | (84) |
| 9. Recipes................................................... | (85) |
| FAQ............................................................ | (93) |
| Epilogue...................................................... | (98) |
| References................................................... | (101) |

## Acknowledgements

This book would not have been possible without the help of my team. First and foremost, I would like to thank my parents, Brad and Jodie Crandall for allowing me to bounce ideas off them at various points in the writing process. They have been incredibly supportive from beginning to end. Next, I would like to thank my editor, Jacob Chester for all the hard-work he put into helping me get this book just right. This man was one of my biggest critics just a year ago but has now joined me in the pursuit of plant-based gains. This tatted, libertarian, motorcycle-riding, beer-drinking, southern boy was one of the last people I would have ever expected to go vegan, but here we are. If he can see the benefits of a plant-based diet, then anyone can. I would also like to sincerely thank the artist who produced the fantastic image on the cover, JohnLee Barnett aka Pancakes. He was able to capture my vision perfectly and help me produce some amazing cover art. Finally, I would like to thank my longtime girlfriend, Rachel Margolis, who puts up with me day in and day out and lived with me during this entire writing process. She helped me develop many of the key ideas in this book, provided me with marketing guidance, and helped me navigate the litigious aspects of writing a book. I will be eternally grateful for the aid all these great people have provided to help me produce this project.

# A Note to Readers

I recognize that any diet runs the risk of being labelled a fad diet and accruing a zealot following of dedicated brainwashed supporters. Unlike many fad diets, the plant-based diet I advocate for in this text is not based on any specific set of strict principles. This is because I recognize that diet is a complex issue and the ideal diet will vary from individual to individual. There is no one size fits all approach to optimizing human health. In the following text, I simply make the argument that most people would stand to benefit from a diet that features plant foods and limits animal foods. I want people to strive towards replacing animal products in their diet with plant-based alternatives. That's it. That's the diet. No pretentious standard needs to be met to be plant-based. All I ask is that people do the best that they honestly can.

I try to limit my discussion of ethics regarding the relation of animal rights and the environment to plant-based diets at any further point in this book. I fear that focusing on these topics will detract from the argument that plant-based diets are beneficial for health, but I will briefly discuss ethics in this prologue, and may lightly mention them later.

Ethics are purely subjective, but there are strong ethical arguments in favor of plant-based diets in addition to the objective health benefits outlined in this book. You don't need to be a hippy animal rights activist to find undeniable cruelty in the way animal agriculture is currently being conducted. Bringing life into this world for the sole purpose of death and profit inevitably leads to immoral behavior. If you're not comfortable watching how animals are treated at factory farms, then you shouldn't be comfortable with supporting the industry.

What makes the life of agricultural animals any less valuable than that of your pets whom most consider family? Cows and pigs experience the same pain and range of emotions that your dog does. My rule of thumb is that if you would not treat your dog the same way you treat a cow or a pig, it is probably wrong.

This book was written for the sole purpose of discussing the benefits to strength training on a plant-based diet. However, I would have serious regrets if I were to fail to discuss the relation of plant-based diets to the state of the world during which this book was written. The following text was written during one of the most severe human health crises in history, the COVID-19 pandemic. So far, this entirely preventable global pandemic has taken more lives than the Vietnam war and the death toll is still rapidly growing as I write. At the moment, the exact origin of this deadly novel coronavirus remains relatively uncertain. Yet, one thing remains clear: this virus was zoonotic in nature and was transferred to humans via the consumption of animals.

This is not the first time humanity has encountered a deadly zoonotic infectious disease. Ebola, SARS, H5N1-Bird Flu, E. Coli, Salmonella, NIPAH, MERS, H7N9-Bird Flu, H1N1-Swine Flu, Mad Cow Disease, and the Seasonal Flu all originated from animal-human contact. Virologists knew that a deadly global pandemic was coming long ago, yet nobody acted appropriately to prevent it. Live animal markets and animal agriculture have exacerbated the potential for deadly diseases to mutate and transfer to humans more than any other factor. If humanity continues to force animals close together in unhygienic environments in close proximity to people for the production of animal products, another deadly pandemic like COVID-19 is inevitable.

It deeply saddens me that instead of making the connection that the large-scale consumption of animals leads to pandemics, the United States has resorted to politicizing the crisis. Rather than working with the world to collectively prevent future pandemics, we have resorted to tribalism and nationalism. Instead of stepping up to the challenge presented by the coronavirus, we place blame on other countries and even fight amongst ourselves. Instead of leaning into science to craft a robust response, we leaned into rhetoric and political narratives. There are many actions that can be taken to help prevent future pandemics from wiping out humanity, but they will all be in vain if animal agriculture is not addressed.

On a similar note, the economic and health damage caused by the novel coronavirus will pale in comparison to that caused by global climate change. The ongoing pandemic during which this book was written has provided the world with a taste of what a global climate crisis may look like. By some estimates, the emissions from animal agriculture are as great as the entire transportation sector. Although systemic change will be needed in many sectors to stop climate change, until emissions reach zero across all sectors, climate change will continue to worsen. This means that there is no slowing climate change without seriously rethinking what we put onto our plate. We need both systemic and individual action to reduce the emissions associated with agriculture. Shifting towards a plant-based diet gives consumers the power to vote with their dollar on an individual level leading to systemic change in the food industry. This brings humanity one step closer towards mitigating a climate catastrophe.

Before you put this book down in an attempt to escape the harsh reality of the modern world, allow me to offer a glimmer of hope. We know what we need to do as a society to treat all beings ethically, stop future global pandemics, and mitigate climate change. We just need to do it. We need to listen to our public health officials, climate scientists, epidemiologists, engineers, nurses, chemists, and environmental scientists. We have the tools available to us to ensure that the planet will be habitable for future generations. Let's use them. I would never argue that a plant-based diet is the fix-all solution to stopping climate change and future global pandemics, but in some cases, making a difference can be as simple as choosing to change the food you put onto your plate. And hey, you might even get stronger and healthier while you're at it.

# Introduction

**M**y education as a chemical engineer has allowed me to develop excellent problem solving and analytical skills. I have applied these skills while working for the Department of Energy at Oak Ridge National Laboratory, the same laboratory that played a key role in the development of the atomic bomb, and while providing technical insight to policy makers in Washington, DC on solutions to climate change.

My approach to solving problems is incredibly trivial: start simple. When chemical engineers approach a complex problem, the very first thing we are trained to do is to make reasonable assumptions that allow the problem to simplified. For example, I may have to assume a certain chemical process is being performed at room temperature if this information is not provided to me.

Non-engineers also make assumptions when they approach problems, they just may not be as aware of these assumptions as an engineer would. The difference between engineers and the general population is that engineers are trained to be incredibly wary of their assumptions since a bad assumption may lead them astray.

The beliefs of the general population are riddled with bad assumptions. One of these bad assumptions is that humans NEED to consume animal products. I too, at one point in time, was personally guilty of this assumption. As a high school senior, I wrote a persuasive essay on "Why you should not go vegan or vegetarian" for my final project in English. If my memory serves me correct, I believe I was awarded a B. Admittedly, this assumption that humans need to consume animals likely had to with my conditioned belief that "meat makes you a man" and insecurities in my own masculinity. I have obviously overcome this insecurity and have become much more educated on nutrition since. It was also awfully convenient for me to believe that I needed to eat meat considering that I enjoyed eating it and derived a sense of masculinity from it.

Coming out of high school, I was recruited to play linebacker at John Carroll University, a small D3 school, but one of the best D3 schools in the country. Most of the attention from the larger schools was absorbed by my high school quarterback, Mitchell Trubisky, the current starting quarterback for the Chicago Bears. Nevertheless, I was thrilled to have the opportunity to play collegiate football at John Carroll given the number of greats they have produced. The late Don Shula, the winningest head coach in NFL history, and Josh McDaniels, the current offensive coordinator for the New England Patriots both played football at John Carroll. In college, I had the chance to train with one of the best strength and conditioning coaches around, Tim Robertson, who has worked with Lebron James, Ted Ginn Jr., and multiple Super Bowl Champions. Even in high school I was surrounded by great coaching in the weight room, working with the strength and conditioning coaches for the Cleveland Indians and Scott Panchik, one of the top competitive crossfitters in the world. Although my collegiate football career was cut short by a fractured spine, I was still given the opportunity to be surrounded by greatness and have witnessed first-hand what it takes to achieve the highest levels of athletic performance.

After a few years of some serious lower back rehabilitation, I was ready to start competing as an athlete again. There was no going back to football at this point, but given my knack for the weight room, I became interested in powerlifting. For those who are unfamiliar, a powerlifting competition consists of three lifts: the squat, the bench, and the deadlift (in that order). Each competitor gets three attempts at the three lifts and the best attempts at each lift are summed to get a total. Whoever has the highest total, wins. A simple competition, but one of the greatest and most objective tests of raw human strength.

In 2019, I competed in my first powerlifting competition in the drug tested division of the American Powerlifting Federation (APF) in the 242 lb. weight class. I did incredibly well and set all the South Carolina state records in the junior class (25 and under) in addition to the state record for the deadlift and the total in the open class (all ages). I squatted 546 lbs., benched 342 lbs., and deadlifted 617 lbs. for a whopping total of 1505 lbs. To the shock of my fellow competitors, I did this all while consuming a diet consisting entirely of plants.

By viewing the body as a machine, I have used my technical background as an engineer to maximize the efficiency of the human diet. Through the lens of my training in chemical engineering, I have concluded that the human organic machine achieves maximal productivity on a predominantly plant-based diet. As a result of this conclusion, I have been able to develop exceptional strength and muscle mass not despite, but because I consume a plant-based diet. In the following text, I hope to share my journey and outline how I achieved high performance using the power of plants. Additionally, I intend to uncover the mechanisms behind potential athletic performance benefits that many plant-based athletes including myself have taken advantage of.

# Chapter 1: The Experiment

**M**y work as a chemical engineer has always revolved around climate change mitigation. Upon arriving to the University of South Carolina, after transferring there following my spinal injury, I began to search for ways I could make an impact. I became involved in research at Carolina in Dr. Jochen Lauterbach's Strategic Approaches to the Generation of Electricity (SAGE) Research Group. This group sought ways to produce energy in a more sustainable manner and I worked for them during my entire undergraduate career on a variety of projects including biofuel production, converting carbon emissions to valuable chemicals, and producing clean hydrogen fuel from water and sunlight.

Somewhere around 2016, I discovered that animal products, especially meat and dairy, are responsible for a significant portion of greenhouse gas emissions. As somebody who sought to mitigate climate change, I felt like a hypocrite for eating such a meat-heavy diet for so long.

The greenhouse gas emissions that result from the production of animal products is roughly equivalent to the entire transportation sector. I am hesitant to provide a firm quantification of the environmental impact of animal agriculture since estimations vary widely, largely due to complexities within the supply chain and lifecycle of animal products. However, if you include the land degradation, air pollution, water shortages, loss of biodiversity, and greenhouse gas emissions associated with the animal agricultural sector, you will find the environmental costs add up quite quickly. If you ascertain nothing else from this book, let it be this: the single best way to personally reduce your environmental impact is to avoid the consumption of animal products.

Energy and the environment are my true areas of expertise. I could probably write an entire book on this topic and may do so one day, but for now, I won't bore you with the details since it is outside the scope of this book. Just know that the environmental degradation caused by animal agriculture causes a great deal of avoidable suffering in the world.

Anyways, upon discovering the environmental impact of animal agriculture back in 2016, I began to transition towards a plant-based vegan diet (a diet void of meat, eggs, and dairy). At the time, it was unclear to me how this would affect my performance in the gym, so I decided to treat this dietary shift as an experiment. I sought to determine the effect of exchanging animal products for plants on my strength, muscle mass, and aesthetic appeal. I made the bad assumption that I wouldn't be able to go all the way vegan without losing my gains, so I decided that I would conduct this experiment in phases to get a better idea of how close I could get to eating a diet that consisted entirely of plants. The first phase would involve the elimination of red meat since this would provide the largest change to my carbon footprint.* This change was easy enough for me to do, given that I mostly consumed leaner white meats like chicken and fish at the time anyways. After about a week or so, I was ready for the next phase of the experiment. The next step was expected to be a little more difficult, the elimination of chicken.

Like many Americans, chicken had been a staple in my diet for as long as I could remember, so taking this leap was intimidating but I was determined to press on. I became pescatarian (only consuming meat from fish along with eggs and dairy). This was probably the most challenging step for me in

---

*As ruminants, cows produce large quantities of methane as a biproduct of digestion. Contrary to popular belief, most of this methane is released out of their mouths not their rear. Methane is a much more powerful greenhouse gas than carbon dioxide, so the beef industry plays a large role in exacerbating global climate change.

the entire process since it required me to seek out new recipes. I could obviously only eat fish, broccoli, and rice so many times before getting sick of it. I also only tried to consume low-mercury fish and consume fish once a day at most since I had developed a justifiable fear of mercury poisoning.[†] I was pescatarian for the largest interval in this experiment because if I was going to lose my gains, I expected it would start at this step. However, I ended up gaining both strength and muscle mass while cutting (eating at a caloric deficit) over the course of summer 2017 while pescatarian. So far, my experiment was going swimmingly, and I had proven to myself that a pescatarian diet would not cause me to shrivel up like many of my friends and family feared.

I was ready for phase 3, removing meat from my diet altogether and becoming vegetarian (only consuming eggs and dairy). This was a big step for me. I had been taught all my life, based on bad assumptions, that meat is what made me strong. I was fully prepared to lose some of my gains for the sake of the experiment at this step and was ready to go back to being pescatarian if I needed to. I paid extra attention to the experiment during this phase and captured weekly progress pictures as shown on the next page and I monitored my performance in the gym closely. Spoiler alert: I thrived as a vegetarian. I was able to gain strength, put on muscle, and intentionally decrease my body fat all at once. After 3 months of being vegetarian, I went from weighing about 225 to 215 lbs. while making improvements on my personal records for the squat, bench, and deadlift. One of the first lifts that tends to suffer from weight loss is the bench press. Three months into vegetarianism, my bench max jumped 10 lbs.

---

[†]Coal-burning power plants have released a significant amount of toxic mercury into the environment that bioaccumulates in fish. Fish towards the top of the food chain like tuna contain the most mercury and pose the greatest health risk. Both the U.S. Food and Drug Administration and the Environmental Protection Agency recommend limiting fish consumption due to potential mercury poisoning.

Day before going
vegetarian

→ More muscle mass

→ Increased strength

→ Decreased body fat

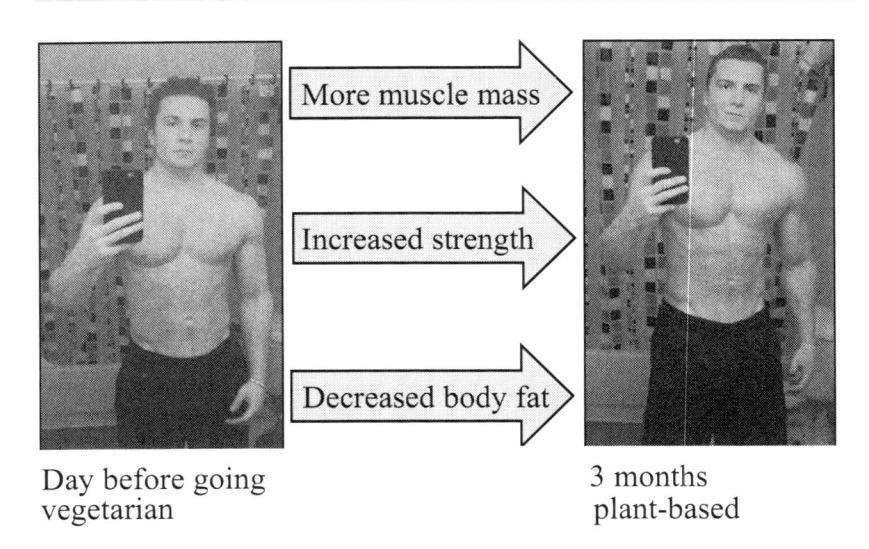

3 months
plant-based

Most people would probably find it easier to first remove eggs then dairy from their diet "because cheese" but I was compelled to remove dairy before the eggs after discovering the emissions associated with dairy are similar to that of beef. This shouldn't really be unexpected since the dairy and beef industries cannot be fully decoupled. What do you think happens to male calves and their mothers after they stop producing milk? In addition to my desire to reduce my carbon footprint as quickly as possible, I have to admit that I have never quite understood the cheese craze. Sure, I enjoyed cheese on pizza and lasagna, but strongly disliked most cheeses outside the realm of parmesan and mozzarella.

At this point in the experiment, I was so determined to get to the final phase that I removed the dairy from my diet and one week later, I was ready to remove the eggs. On top of that, my roommate at the time had been inspired by my experiment to go fully vegan (refraining from using all animal products) cold turkey, so of course I couldn't fall short at this point. When people go vegan cold turkey, they often report remarkable changes such as increases in energy or their skin clearing up. Personally, since my transition was so gradual, I didn't notice any significant instantaneous physical changes, but I certainly felt better as a vegan than when I had started the experiment. My sex drive had gone through the roof, I was sleeping better, and felt that I had more energy throughout the day. I actually expected to feel worse after transitioning to veganism so this was a pleasant surprise for me. These effects could very well be attributed to some type of reverse placebo effect, but are worth mentioning, nonetheless.

Not only did I feel better as a result of removing animal products from my diet, my performance in the gym also improved. I was getting stronger noticeably faster and my recovery time decreased significantly. I was able to move more weight and be less sore the next day which is a HUGE advantage in any athletic endeavor. If you can do more damage to the muscles of the body and then recover from that damage more rapidly, you have a huge edge over your competitors. I'll get into the mechanism behind the muscle recovery benefits on a plant-based diet a little later in the book.

As a scientist, I would be remiss if I failed to point out that this "experiment" I carried out on myself was obviously not a scientifically validated study. It shouldn't be treated as anything other than an anecdote. This research would never make it past peer review for an academic journal, but I never intended to add to the body of academic knowledge with my project. My experiment was conducted out of pure curiosity to find the most sustainable diet I could personally consume without seeing a significant decrease in my muscle mass and strength. The discovery of potential performance benefits was simply the side product of this pursuit. If I am being completely honest, I had very little faith this experiment would go well. I expected that at some point during the transition, my muscle mass would simply begin to atrophy. I did not have a good explanation as to why I thought my muscles would atrophy, this was just what I had been conditioned all my life to believe. On the contrary to my preconceived notions, my personal athletic performance thrived on a fully vegan plant-based diet. As it turns out, I was not the only athlete to make this discovery…

# Chapter 2: The Next Generation of Elite Athletes

From Tom Brady to Serena Williams, the world's top athletes all seem to be slowly realizing the power of plant-based diets. Brady, the six-time super bowl champion and Serena, the 22-time grand slam champion have both already recognized the benefits of a plant-based diet. Serena and Venus Williams have been eating a nearly completely vegan diet since around 2012 when Venus was diagnosed with Sjögren's syndrome, an autoimmune disease, and advised by her doctor to remove animal products from her diet. In the world of men's tennis, Novak Djokovic has also adopted a plant-based diet and even opened his own vegan restaurant.

Tom Brady reportedly consumes a vegan diet nearly year-round to minimize inflammation. Brady has even partnered with vegan meal delivery service Purple Carrot and sells his own line of TB12 vegan snacks. Brady's diet has had a profound influence on record breaking tight end and fellow teammate Rob Gronkowski who reportedly adopted a predominately plant-based diet back in 2017. In addition to Gronkowski, fellow legendary NFL quarterback, Aaron Rodgers of the Green Bay Packers was also influenced by Tom Brady to consume a predominantly plant-based diet. Rodgers has eliminated dairy from his diet and claims that about 80% of his meals are now vegan. None of these athletes mentioned have adopted an incredibly strict vegan diet, but each of them avoids consuming animal products and derives nearly all their calories from plants so most of them are close to being fully vegan.

Since the athletes listed above do consume small amounts of animal products from time to time, critics may argue that this occasional indulgence is the source of their strength and energy. This argument is easily weakened by the plethora of 100% vegan athletes, some of whom have been vegan for decades or even their entire life. Look no further than documentaries like James Cameron's and Arnold Schwarzenegger's *The Gamechangers* or *From The Ground Up* to catch a glimpse into the world of vegan athletes. These documentaries boast about vegan strength athletes such as Germany's Strongest Man, Patrik Baboumian and Olympic Weightlifter, Kendrick Farris who was the only male USA weightlifter to qualify for the 2016 Rio Olympics. Professional bodybuilders, Nimai Delgado (NPC Men's Physique National Champion/IFBB Pro) and Barny Du Plessis (Mr. Universe 2014) have also received international recognition for their plant-fueled strength.

In addition to strength athletes, UFC fighter, Nate Diaz and nine-time gold winning Olympic sprinter, Carl Lewis have also thrived on plant-based diets. Besides Brady and Gronk on Patriots, about 15 players on the Tennessee Titans have adopted plant-based diets thanks to Chef Charity Morgan who provides them with delicious vegan meals. Veganism seems to be getting a lot of traction in the NFL lately with stars such as Cam Newton, Colin Kaepernick, Tyrann Mathiu and many others also going vegan.

Even the NBA is getting on the plant-based train with athletes such as Kyrie Irving, Damian Lillard, Jahlil Okafor, Wilson Chandler and many more adopting plant-based diets to varying degrees. In the realm of powerlifting, vegan athletes such as International Powerlifting League (IPL) World Champion, Nick Squires, IPL World Championship runner-up and author of *The Way of the Vegan Meathead*, Daniel Austin, and myself are also making waves. Everywhere you look now has elite plant-based athletes. Soccer has Lionel Messi, hockey has Stanley Cup champion and Boston Bruins captain, Zdeno Chara. Ultramarathoning has a plethora of athletes including one of the most dominant runners in the world, Scott Jurek. Major League Baseball has two-time all-star pitcher Pat Neshek along with World Series champion pitcher Carsten Charles Sabathia. The list goes on and on.

Even with the impressive roster that I have listed, fully vegan plant-based athletes still represent a minority of all athletes. It should be noted that vegans make up a small, but rapidly growing portion of the world's total population. With that said, the percentage of elite athletes adopting plant-based diets appears to be growing much more rapidly than in the general population. Even the athletes that are unwilling to go completely vegan, are significantly reducing animal product consumption. This forces one to conclude that either plant-based diets are propelling athletes to the world stage or that world stage athletes are increasingly adopting plant-based diets. Either way, this is a strong testament to the power of plants and this phenomenon is probably worth exploring.

# Chapter 3: The Plant-Based Edge

I have sufficiently demonstrated a trend towards plant-based diets in all types of athletics. The fundamental question I have yet to answer in detail is why have these athletes chosen to adopt and stick to plant-based diets? I seriously doubt that this many world-class athletes are now avoiding animal products for fun or to simply participate in a new trend. Therefore, the athletes I have listed must have recognized some benefit to consuming a diet featuring plants. A ground-breaking study published in 2020 explored the trend towards plant-based diets amongst athletes.[1] The study compared a group of vegan college athletes with omnivorous college athletes and found that the vegans achieved a better exercise performance. Why is that? In this chapter I will attempt to answer that question and identify the principal benefits to consuming a diet void of animal products.

Portions of this chapter will be speculative, but I will do my best to back up my claims with as much evidence as possible. Unfortunately, since widespread veganism amongst athletes is a relatively recent movement, the plant-based edge has yet to be completely fleshed out in the world of nutrition science. With that said, I have personally concluded that a diet completely void of animal products provides an edge in athletic performance. Contrary to commonly held beliefs, this edge seems particularly prevalent when it comes to strength sports. I may not be able to successfully convince you of this, but I hope that after reading this chapter you will understand why I have made such a bold statement. At the very least, I hope you will recognize that plant-based athletes certainly face no competitive disadvantages due to their diet.

## Increased Micronutrient Intake

First and foremost, possibly the single greatest advantage that plant-based athletes have in comparison to their omnivorous competitors is the fact that they likely consume more micronutrients. In other words, they're consuming more vitamins and minerals which play a vital role in a wide variety of critical processes in the human body. It is impossible to supplement all these micronutrients and achieve the same results due to absorption issues. Additionally, it is likely that we have yet to identify the importance of many micronutrients and would have no way of knowing to supplement them.

I understand there is likely some skepticism about my claim that vegans consume more micronutrients than meat-eaters. However, this shouldn't be a shocking revelation considering that the original source of all micronutrients in animal-based foods are plant-based foods. As you move up the food chain, some of the micronutrients from the original plant-based source may be concentrated, but most are lost so it is beneficial to consume micronutrients directly from the bottom of the food chain.

Please allow me to elaborate upon the idea that plant-based foods are more micronutrient dense than animal-based foods with a few examples. We'll start with an easy example. Consider milk. Let's examine the micronutrient content of 2% dairy milk and soymilk on the next page. We'll equalize the calories to 138 (1 serving/1 cup of 2% dairy milk) to keep this comparison as fair as possible:

| Micronutrient | 2% Dairy Milk (%DV) | Soymilk (%DV) |
|---|---|---|
| Vitamin A | 0% | 28% |
| Vitamin B12 | 60% | 215% |
| Vitamin C | 0% | 0% |
| Vitamin D | 22% | 34% |
| Vitamin E | 0% | 0% |
| Vitamin K | 0% | 0% |
| Fiber | 0% | 9% |
| Calcium | 33% | 51% |
| Iron | 0% | 23% |
| Magnesium | 7% | 17% |
| Potassium | 11% | 17% |
| Zinc | 12% | 0% |

*Data obtained from Cronometer

If you thought that you needed to drink cow's milk to build strong bones, then guess again! Soymilk has significantly more calcium and vitamin D than dairy milk. I know what you're thinking, "But cow's milk has more protein!" Wrong again. I wanted to only focus on the micronutrients in the table above, so I didn't list protein, but soymilk has more protein than cow's milk. Soymilk has 12 g of protein per 138 calories, whereas 2% dairy milk has a measly 9 g of protein per 138 calories.

It was a shocking revelation for me when I first discovered that the micronutrient content of soymilk is superior to that of dairy milk. Yet again one of the false assumptions that society had led me to believe about animal product consumption turned out to be wrong. This false assumption is likely the result of the incredibly successful "Got Milk?" ad campaign funded by the dairy industry to deceive the general public. If strong bones are your goal, then you're doing yourself a disservice by consuming dairy milk instead of soymilk.

I know some people may still be skeptical so let's do another comparison. This time we'll compare tofu (delicious when properly prepared) with skinless chicken breast. The following table shows the micronutrient profile of 100 calories of each:

| Micronutrient | Skinless Chicken Breast (%DV) | Tofu (%DV) |
|---|---|---|
| Vitamin A | 0% | 3% |
| Vitamin B12 | 8% | 0% |
| Vitamin C | 0% | 0% |
| Vitamin D | 0% | 0% |
| Vitamin E | 0% | 0% |
| Vitamin K | 0% | 0% |
| Fiber | 0% | 4% |
| Calcium | 0% | 47% |
| Iron | 7% | 23% |
| Magnesium | 3% | 10% |
| Potassium | 4% | 4% |
| Zinc | 6% | 9% |

*Data obtained from Cronometer

Again, it appears that the plant-based option is the clear victor. The tofu wins on every micronutrient compared except vitamin B12. If it isn't starting to become clear at this point that plant foods tend to be more micronutrient dense than animal foods, I'm not sure what will convince you. I did my best to make these comparisons as fair as possible and to not cherry pick. I'm sure there is some comparison out there where an animal food could be shown to be more micronutrient dense, but this is generally not the case. Nearly all plant-based replacements for animal products are typically superior in terms of micronutrient content.

There are many comparisons like the milk and chicken/tofu comparison made above that demonstrate the micronutrient superiority of plant foods. At this point you may assert that you can just add vegetables to an animal-based diet to make up for the micronutrient difference between a plant-based and animal-based diet. To demonstrate the problem with this argument, it's helpful to view daily caloric intake as a caloric budget.

For sake of argument let's assume you have a caloric budget of 2,000 calories. You could spend half of these calories on animal-based foods and the other half on plant-based foods OR you could spend all 2,000 of these calories on more nutrient dense plant-based foods. The first approach represents adding vegetables as a side to your steak. The second approach represents a plant-based diet. Sure, the first approach still gives you some micronutrient dense plant food, but the second approach gives you twice as much. I'll demonstrate the vast micronutrient difference between a plant-based meal and an animal-based meal by comparing a meal consisting of a tofu steak with broccoli, buttered (vegan butter) potato, and soymilk to a meal consisting of skinless chicken breast with broccoli, buttered (dairy butter) potato, and 2% dairy milk below:

| Micronutrient | Animal-Based Meal (%DV) | Plant-Based Meal (%DV) |
|---|---|---|
| Vitamin A | **109%** | 105% |
| Vitamin B12 | 71% | **112%** |
| Vitamin C | 131% | 131% |
| Vitamin D | 20% | 20% |
| Vitamin E | 26% | **28%** |
| Vitamin K | 187% | 187% |
| Fiber | 23% | **35%** |
| Calcium | 40% | **133%** |
| Iron | 52% | **96%** |
| Magnesium | 34% | **50%** |
| Potassium | 58% | 58% |
| Zinc | **35%** | 31% |

In addition to the micronutritional differences between the animal-based and plant-based meal shown above, the plant-based meal is also lower in cholesterol, rich in antioxidants, lower in saturated fat, and contains zero hormones. Where the animal-based meal is richer in micronutrients (vitamin A and zinc), it isn't by much. A negligible difference of 4% in both cases. In contrast, where the plant-based meal is richer in micronutrients (vitamin B12, vitamin E, fiber, calcium, iron, magnesium, and potassium), the difference is much more significant.

A plant-based diet is about spending all or almost all your caloric budget on nutrient-rich plants instead of animal products. It's about replacing dairy milk with more nutrient-rich soymilk and replacing chicken breast with micronutrient packed tofu. It's easy to see that when each animal product in your diet is swapped out for a plant-based alternative, the additional micronutrients add up quickly. These added micronutrients are likely to make a big difference in your exercise performance, recovery, and overall health.

**Decreased Consumption of Junk Food**

Take a moment to think about some of the worst foods you can put into your body. Things like ice cream, donuts, hot dogs, fried chicken, and cake will likely come to mind. What do all these foods have in common? They are loaded with animal products. By committing to a plant-based diet, these foods are automatically off the table. This makes dealing with the temptation much easier. Somebody who is simply tracking calories will be more tempted by these foods and will be able to convince themselves that they'll make these junk foods fit into their caloric budget or just work off the calories later. This excuse doesn't work so well when you have committed to a plant-based diet because these products aren't plant-based. No amount of mental gymnastics will convince you that you can have just a few bites of these tempting animal-based junk foods.

Some people may argue that with the advent of more vegan fast food options that vegans will be just as tempted as their omnivorous peers. This is somewhat true, but it fails to account for the fact that the plant-based versions of animal-based junk foods are almost always healthier. I'm not going to advocate for consuming an entire diet based on impossible whoppers, but at the end of the day, you're much better off eating these plant-based patties than the original beef whopper. Still skeptical? Let's take a closer look at the original whopper and the impossible whopper. The table below compares the nutritional content of an impossible burger patty with that of a 70-90% lean beef burger patty:

|  | **Impossible Beef** | **70-90% Lean Beef** |
| --- | --- | --- |
| Weight | 113 g | 113 g |
| Calories | 240 | 235-305 |
| Protein | 19 g | 17-28 g |
| Fat | 17 g | 12-20 g |
| Carbs | 7 g | 0 g |
| Trans Fat | **0 g** | 1 g |
| Saturated Fat | 8 g | 7-8 g |
| Cholesterol | **0 mg** | 100 mg |
| Vitamin B12 | **130%** | 48-130% |
| Vitamin B1 | **2350%** | 4% |
| Vitamin B2 | **30%** | 12% |
| Fiber | **3 g** | 0 g |
| Folate | **30%** | 4% |
| Calcium | **170 mg** | 8 mg |
| Zinc | **50%** | 41-48% |
| Iron | **4.2 mg** | 3 mg |
| Selenium | 0% | **35%** |
| Antioxidants | **Higher** | Lower |
| Hormones | **No** | Yes |

*Data obtained from Cronometer

Note: Information on important nutrients like vitamin C and D are missing because Impossible Foods has not provided that information for their impossible beef.

Just a quick glance at this data reveals the nutritional superiority of an impossible burger over a beef burger. Even if the beef is 90% lean, which is an incredibly generous assumption for a whopper, the impossible burger still comes out on top. An impossible burger contains many of the nutrients that the body needs like vitamin B12, B1, B2, fiber, folate, calcium, iron, and antioxidants. A beef burger contains things like trans-fat, cholesterol, and hormones that are harmful to the body. One may argue that the beef patty may contain more protein, but that's only if the beef is incredibly lean. Most beef burgers are much closer to 70% lean than 90% lean. When this is considered, the protein content of the two types of burgers appears to be about the same. I refuse to place a positive or negative connotation upon the macronutrients (protein, carbs, and fat) because everyone's macronutritional needs are different. Finally, the caloric content of the two burgers appears similar with the beef burger probably being slightly higher in calories than the impossible burger. Again, I refuse to assign a positive or negative connotation to calories because if you're bulking more calories are desirable, whereas when you're cutting, fewer calories are desirable. I cannot assume that calories are inherently good nor bad.

With that said, I do acknowledge that there are a lot of junk food vegans out there, but those on a plant-based diet are far less likely to consume these empty calorie foods. When they do splurge and consume junk food, it is still a plant-based food which is typically healthier than animal-based junk food. This accompanies the previously discussed idea that plant-based diets are more micronutrient dense than animal-based diets.

**Improved Microbiome**

While easily overlooked, the plumbing, or digestive system of the living machine is critical to maximizing performance in the body. Research has overwhelmingly demonstrated that plant-based diets promote helpful gut bacteria in the intestines.[2] This gut bacteria makes up what is referred to as the "microbiome";

micro meaning small and biome meaning community. The possession of a healthy microbiome is critical for a wide variety of functions in the human body. One of the most important of these functions for a lifter is the ability of the microbiome to destroy compounds called antinutrients that prevent mineral absorption. These pesky antinutrients can rob the body of consumed nutrients needed for recovery. Plant-based diets help get rid of these antinutrients.

It has been argued that since plant-based diets are typically higher in legumes that contain antinutrients like lectins and phytates, those on plant-based diets may increase their consumption of antinutrients. This is a misleading assertion that has been perpetuated by pseudoscientific fad dieters like the author of *The Plant Paradox*. The reality is that shelling, soaking, and cooking legumes virtually eliminates all these antinutrients.[3,4] Unless you're regularly consuming uncooked beans, you have absolutely nothing to worry about.

The fad dieters that fear monger about legumes are often the same fad dieters pushing low fiber diets.[‡] The inherently high fiber content of a plant-based diet is what is mostly behind the enhanced microbiome of those on plant-based diets. Only about 5% of Americans consume enough fiber, but most people on a plant-based diet have no problem consuming enough fiber.[5] I routinely consume more than double, sometimes triple, my recommend daily fiber intake.

Fiber is so important that many bodybuilders and powerlifters use it as a metric to quantify diet quality. This is for a good reason. Increased fiber intake has been found to lower risk for developing coronary heart disease, stroke, hypertension,

---

[‡]There appears to be a troubling increase in people promoting high meat diets such as carnivore and keto. The lack of fiber in these diets alone should be enough to dissuade anybody with a good head on their shoulders from giving them a try. Do not be fooled by the outrageous claims made by these meat pushing zealots. These diets have the potential to pose a serious health risk due to lack of fiber.

diabetes, obesity, and certain gastrointestinal diseases while decreasing blood pressure and reducing blood cholesterol.[6] If fiber intake starts dropping, my fellow meathead colleagues know that the quality of their food sources is low.

Here's the kicker: there is absolutely zero fiber found in animal products. Fiber is found exclusively in plants. If my omnivorous lifter colleagues are going to use fiber as a diet quality metric, wouldn't it logically follow that the highest quality diet is one void of animal products? It seems to me that the easiest way to maximize fiber intake and diet quality would be to consume a plant-based diet. When my fellow lifters use fiber as a metric for diet quality, they're really using whole plant food consumption to measure diet quality. I'd go so far as to argue that fiber could just be a proxy for measuring the amount of whole plant foods people are eating. Meaning that many of the benefits we attribute to increased fiber intake could potentially just be the benefits of eating more quality unprocessed plant foods and fewer animal products.

A big issue many people have when they first adopt a plant-based diet is that they feel bloated. Do not be alarmed. This is the result of getting your fiber intake to where it should be. Bloating should subside within a few weeks at most once the microbiome has a chance to adjust to all the fiber it was previously lacking. If the bloating is particularly bothersome, I would suggest slowly ramping up fiber intake. Track how much fiber you eat each day and increase it by 10 g at first. Once you are comfortable, increase it by another 10 g, and so on until you feel like you are eating a comfortable ratio of whole to processed plant foods that works for you (whole plant foods are typically much higher in fiber than processed plant foods).

**Faster Recovery**

Many people that believe they are overtraining are simply under recovering. One of the most important factors that promotes success in top tier athletes is the quality of their recovery between training sessions. Ultimately, the athlete that can recover quicker can train more. The entire premise behind strength training is to tear down the body so it can be built back up and become stronger. You have a significant advantage over your competition if you can tear down and build up more rapidly than them. This is one of the many advantages offered by a plant-based diet.

Inflammation and oxidative stress can severely impair muscle recovery. A little inflammation is good and is a natural response to heal the body. However, this inflammation can linger even after the body is repaired damaging healthy muscles and joints.[7] This unnecessary inflammation can be promoted by the consumption of inflammatory compounds found in food leading to negative impacts on physical performance.[8]

Some of the most inflammatory compounds for the human body are found in animal products. Compounds such as the carnitine found in animal tissue causes the body to produce a chemical called trimethlyamine oxide (TMAO) that can stimulate inflammation.[9] On top of TMAO, another inflammatory compound called heme iron is found in large quantities in animal products. Heme iron concentrations are especially high in red meat and processed meat. The consumption of a single hamburger has been shown to increase inflammation by 70%.[10] This is because the body has a very difficult time regulating how quickly heme iron is absorbed. When heme iron is consumed, the body becomes flooded with more iron than it can handle, leading to inflammation.[11] Heme iron is a different type of iron than the iron found in plant foods. The nonheme iron in plant foods does not overwhelm the body as easily, decreasing the risk for inflammation. I'll discuss this more later in the book in Chapter 7.

The high concentration of heme iron found in meat is part of the reason why the World Health Organization (WHO) has classified red meat (beef, pork, lamb, veal, etc.) as a Group 2A carcinogen (probably cancer causing) and has classified processed meat (beef jerky, bacon, hot dogs, ham, etc.) as a

Group 1 carcinogen (causes cancer).[12] For a frame of reference, cigarettes are also classified as a Group 1 carcinogen by the WHO. However, this does not necessarily mean smoking a pack of cigarettes is the same thing as eating a sausage. The effects are different, but the WHO is just as confident that processed meat can cause cancer as they are that cigarettes cause cancer. In fact, they found that each 50 g portion of processed consumed daily increases the risk of colorectal cancer by 18%.[12] This is a strong enough reason to avoid the consumption of processed meat without even considering the negative impacts on strength training due to inflammation.

In addition to TMAO and heme iron, saturated fat has also been found to induce inflammation.[13] Saturated fat is found in meat, dairy, eggs as well as tropical oils like coconut and palm oil. However, those on a plant-based diet typically consume very little saturated fat since most saturated fat is primarily found in animal products.[14]

Not only do those on a plant-based diet avoid the consumption of inflammatory compounds like heme iron, TMAO, and saturated fat, they also consume more antioxidants. These antioxidants help prevent inflammation in the body from occurring in the first place, improving recovery speed. This is the entire premise of Tom Brady's TB12 plant-based diet. On average, plants contain 64 times more antioxidants than animal products.[15] This means that even if you only eat a little meat, you are missing out on the antioxidants you could be consuming if you were eating entirely plant-based. You are spending some of your caloric budget on inflammatory meat instead of antioxidant rich plant foods.

A recent study had participants adopt a plant-based vegan diet and within only three weeks, inflammation dropped by a whopping 29%.[16] How does this translate to strength training? A large body of research has shown that an increased antioxidant intake directly leads to reduced muscle damage, decreased soreness, and the promotion of recovery.[17–21] All of these factors contribute to improved performance by allowing the body to build itself up more rapidly between training sessions. This allows a lifter to train harder and more often. Ultimately, training harder and more often over time is what separates the good athletes from the great.

When it comes down to it, the difference between the elite lifter and the average lifter is that the elite simply put more work in. An antioxidant rich, plant-based diet free of inflammatory compounds found in animal products is no magic pill that will get you shredded overnight. Brendan Brazier, pro ironman triathlete and cofounder of Vega, once said, "Being vegan doesn't make you a stronger, better athlete. But it allows you to make yourself a stronger, better athlete." A plant-based diet simply puts a lifter in a position to maximize the amount of work that can be achieved by the human body. To take full advantage of this increased work capacity requires pushing yourself beyond what you were previously capable of. However, once this work capacity is increased, the gains will follow at an accelerated rate. If that doesn't get you excited, then this book probably isn't for you.

**Enhanced Blood Flow**

The living machine's circulatory system is analogous to that of a complex system of pipes in a chemical plant. This internal piping directs oxygen throughout the body via an organic pump, the heart. If this internal piping becomes clogged, it impedes nutrient flow and oxygen transport which decreases the efficiency of the living machine. The buildup of cholesterol plaque in human arteries can cause this type of clogging. This is disastrous for a lifter because it means less oxygen reaches your muscles.

One of the benefits of an entirely plant-based diet related to blood flow that I cannot emphasize enough is the elimination of dietary cholesterol. There is absolutely zero cholesterol in plant foods, it is found exclusively in animal products. If you're vegan and are consuming a product with cholesterol in it, you better double check the ingredients. Some animal foods like eggs are especially high in cholesterol. In fact, two eggs have more cholesterol (372 mg) in them than the daily recommended cholesterol intake (300 mg). It is easy to see how quickly cholesterol can add up when you're consuming animal products every meal.

In addition to preventing the internal piping from becoming clogged from cholesterol, plant-based diets can also increase the flow rate of blood into muscle tissue. The circulatory system can be thought of as an oxygen delivery service. This means more oxygen can be delivered to your muscles in less time if the blood is flowing more rapidly into muscle tissue. Research has shown that plant-based diets achieve this by decreasing the resistance to flow, or viscosity, of the blood.[22-24]

Viscosity is a physical property that a chemical engineer is familiar with, but rarely encountered by the general public. An example of a fluid with high viscosity would be honey because it is resistant to flow and an example of a fluid with low viscosity is water because it is not very resistant to flow. Plant-based diets decrease blood viscosity making your blood less like honey and more like water. This is desirable because the easier the blood flows, the easier it is to get oxygen to your muscles during a workout. Research has demonstrated that high blood viscosity leads to decreased athletic performance and low blood viscosity, like that achieved on a plant-based diet, leads directly to increased athletic performance.[22,25,26]

Plant-based diets can decrease the viscosity of the blood and prevent the internal piping from clogging, but how does this diet impact your heart which is responsible for pumping the blood around the body? From a purely engineering perspective, the heart is simply a pump and the blood is simply a fluid. I won't bore you with the math behind this, but it is well understood by engineers that fluids with a high viscosity (fluids that resist flow) reduce pump efficiency. I have already explained how plant-based diets decrease the viscosity of the blood which results in oxygen getting to the muscle quicker, but this also has positive impacts on the heart. Highly viscous, honey-like blood takes a big toll on the heart by reducing the efficiency of this organic pump. The heart prefers water-like blood with a low viscosity that can be obtained through a plant-based diet.

Considering that heart disease is the leading cause of death in the U.S., maintaining the heart is critical for human health.[27] Research has shown for years that plant-based diets significantly improve heart health and in turn, increase the lifespan of the entire living machine. When the American Heart Association looked at the entire body of research conducted between 1987-2016, they found that plant-based diets are associated with a lower risk of cardiovascular disease and all-cause mortality.[28]

An old adage in the world of lifting goes something like, "he/she who lifts the longest is the strongest." Any lifter who has suffered a serious injury can attest to the truth of this adage. It takes a long time to build up a solid foundation of muscle mass and strength. It is truly a shame that many lifters lose all those hard-earned gains due to poor health. If you take good care of your body, especially that critical pump that is the literal heart of the entire system, you can steadily make gains while those around you fall victim to illness and injury as their health declines. The benefits of taking care of the heart also obviously extend well beyond the gym. I think everyone would love to see their kids grow old and still be able to feel 40 in their late 60s. This is the type of edge that can be gained via a plant-based diet.

One important bodily function that heavily relies upon good blood flow in males is their ability to achieve erections. There is some limited evidence that suggests plant-based diets may improve male erections. Studies directly examining the effect of a plant-based diet on erectile dysfunction are still ongoing, so I won't jump to any substantive conclusions here yet. However, one researcher has collected some promising preliminary results and others have revealed some interesting findings. Dr. Aaron Spitz, MD, urology specialist and author of *The Penis Book* revealed to the general public in the *Gamechangers* film that he has collected preliminary results demonstrating that a diet void of animal products can lead to stronger, longer lasting erections. Dr. Sptiz's study is still underway, and these preliminary results should be taken with a grain of salt since they haven't been peer-reviewed, but certainly these early results show that this study is worth conducting. I eagerly await the results.

Conclusions cannot be drawn from these preliminary results, but there are studies that indirectly support the idea that a plant-based diet could improve male erections. I have already shown that it is well-understood that plant-based diets can improve cardiovascular health and studies have shown that improved cardiovascular health is associated with decreased erectile dysfunction.[29,30] Plant-based diets lead to good cardiovascular health, which leads to good blood flow, and good blood flow leads to good erections. It would be a bit of a logical jump to suggest that plant-based diets decrease erectile dysfunction based on this information alone, but other studies also seem to point to this idea.

One study found a 10% reduction in erectile dysfunction with each additional serving of fruits and vegetables consumed.[31] It would seem to me that the best way to eat the maximum servings of fruits and vegetables would be on a plant-based diet. Another study found that a higher habitual intake of flavonoids, a compound only found in plant-foods, leads to a reduced incidence of erectile dysfunction.[32] Again, the best way to maximize flavonoid intake is with a plant-based diet.

Overall, I am not willing to strongly conclude that plant-based diets improve erections based on this limited evidence. However, there does seem to be evidence to strongly support that hypothesis. I know that probably just sounds like scientist gibberish to most readers so let me put it more simply. If the question is do plant-based diets lead to better erections? Then the answer is probably, but nobody can say for sure yet. What can be said for sure is that plant-based diets improve blood flow, decrease blood viscosity, promote cardiovascular health and that all these things will be helpful in your pursuit of gains.

**The Chip on the Shoulder Effect**

The final edge granted to the plant-based athlete is not a physiological edge, but a psychological edge. I promise you that long-term vegans are some of the most mentally strong people that you will ever encounter. These are people that have rebelled against the status quo for a higher purpose whether it be to protect the environment, fight for animal rights, improve health, or all the above. Standing up for yourself while constantly being beat down by the world around you takes real guts.

Those of you who have never adopted a plant-based diet may think I'm exaggerating, but it's important for me to let you know what you're in for. The number one reason people don't stick with a plant-based diet is social pressure. It is likely that there are people you are currently close with that will scoff at you for adopting a plant-based diet and berate you for this personal decision. Prior to going vegan my first response to those adopting plant-based diets was certainly quite negative.

Plant-based diets get a bad reputation. Sometimes deservingly so, but usually this is not the case. When you explain your new plant-based diet to somebody who is not plant-based, they will typically feel guilty for not adopting a plant-based themselves. Unfortunately, sometimes this can grow into resentment. People will quickly develop the sense that you feel superior to them for being vegan or vegetarian and will feel the need to justify why they are not plant-based. People will tell you that there is no way to get strong on a plant-based diet or that they need to eat meat. They will suggest that plant-based diets are not conducive to strength training by saying they are feminizing or don't contain enough protein. Personally, I find nothing more motivating than these unpleasant encounters. THIS is what I refer to as the "chip on the shoulder effect."

I encourage you to seek out the doubters around you. They will give you something to prove. These people are typically difficult to persuade so don't waste too much energy trying to convince them. A verbal debate about plant-based diets is usually a lost cause, especially if the conversation is about ethics. There are only three things you need to do during these unpleasant encounters. First, direct them to this book so they can see for themselves why their preconceived notions of plant-based diets are false. (If you're one of these people, congratulations on making it this far!) Second, internalize every word you are told by those who doubt you. Third, and most importantly, go prove them wrong! No matter how much somebody may doubt your ability to build strength and muscle from plants, there is no arguing with real results. As a powerlifter, I have found that the best way to shut somebody's mouth is to get stronger than them. No verbal argument is more powerful than that.

The two strongest motivators in this world are love and hate. Find a reason to love your plant-based diet. It could be the health benefits, the decreased carbon footprint, or the promotion of animal rights. It doesn't matter which of these motivate you. However, it is important for you to have a strong reason for this lifestyle change because it makes the transition so much easier when you have a cause to fall back on when things get tough. I would never encourage you to develop hatred for another human being, but I do encourage you develop a hatred for an idea held by your fellow human beings. Take something negative that you read online or from a conversation about plant-based diets and use it to light a fire in your belly. Once you have identified a source of love and hate, the chip on the shoulder effect will be in full swing. Fueled by the strongest motivators in the world, you are now on your way to making some serious gains.

# Chapter 4: Protein

What most people don't realize prior to adopting a plant-based diet is that it's easy to meet your daily protein needs with plants. Protein can be found in relatively large quantities not only in animal-based foods, but also in plants. Despite what you may have been led to believe, there aren't any protein deficient vegans or vegetarians out there if they're consuming enough calories. Protein deficiency may be the biggest criticism of a plant-based diet, but you will soon see that plants have all the protein that you need. Which begs the question, how much protein do we really need?

## How Much Do I Need?

This is the question that has plagued bodybuilding forums for as long as I have been alive. Everyone with a desire to get bigger and stronger wants to know how much protein they should be eating to accomplish their strength goals. One thing that prevents them from obtaining this knowledge is the rampant rise of a mindless cult of broscientists. Don't be fooled by the name, these people are the antithesis of a scientist. Rather than sourcing information from the peer reviewed scientific literature, they rely upon unreliable anecdotal evidence that is transferred by word of mouth in gym locker rooms. Broscientists seem to be constantly increasing the recommended daily protein intake every year. This is based upon the notion that it is better to overconsume than to under-consume protein. This has some truth to it, but keep in mind that by increasing protein intake, carbohydrate and/or fat intake will need to decrease to maintain a constant caloric intake. Basically, increasing protein intake too much can cost your body the much-needed energy sources it relies upon. There is a careful balance that must be achieved to optimize the living machine.

The most up-to-date protein recommendations for maximizing muscle protein synthesis (MPS) in athletes fall within the range of 1.3-1.8 g/kg (0.6-0.8 g/lb.) each day.[33] This means on average it is recommend that about 1.5 g of protein should be consumed per kg lean body mass each day or about 0.7 g per pound of lean body mass. When studies recommend protein intake in terms of g/kg, broscientists often mistake this notation to mean grams of protein per kilogram of *bodyweight*. In reality, the g/kg notation refers to grams of protein per kilogram of *lean body mass*. The difference between bodyweight and lean body mass is that lean body mass does not account for fat. Lean body mass is a measure of everything in the body besides fat so lean body mass is always lower than bodyweight. Confusing a protein recommendation based on lean body mass for a protein recommendation based on bodyweight is partly what leads to the inflation of protein recommendations you see online. Some broscientists have even taken the recommendation of 1.5 g of protein per lean kg body mass to mean eating 1.5 g of protein per pound bodyweight. Not only has lean body mass been confused for bodyweight, but kilograms have also been confused for pounds. The broscientist recommendation of 1.5 g of protein per pound bodyweight is vastly different from the protein recommendations supported by academic literature.

According to the scientific literature, 1.8-2.0 grams of protein per kilogram lean body mass (0.8-0.9 g/lb.) is recommended each day during training periods of high frequency/intensity.[33] To make the math easier, I'm going to round this up to 1 g/lb. daily (there I go inflating again). Jokes aside, I have a good reason for rounding this up. These daily protein intake recommendations are based upon studies performed on omnivores. Typically, plant-based protein takes a little longer to absorb into the bloodstream because the carbohydrates surrounding it can slow down absorption. Luckily, studies have shown this can be easily accounted for by slightly increasing plant-based protein intake.[34] Let's look at an example of how to apply this rounded protein recommendation: say you weigh 200 lbs. and have 15% body fat, then your lean body mass is 170 lbs. Apply the protein recommendation to this lean body mass, and you should be eating around 170 g of protein per day. If this is too confusing, I've provided a simple formula below:

$$\left(1 - \frac{\text{Body Fat \%}}{100}\right) \times \text{Body Weight} = \text{Daily Protein Intake (in grams)}$$

If you don't know your body fat percentage, make an educated guess. The healthy body fat percentage for men is typically around 15% and for women, around 25%. If you're unfamiliar with body fat percentages, the U.S. Navy has a simple method to calculate it that you can google. All you'll need is a measuring tape and a calculator. This number really doesn't have to be exact so if you're in ballpark range, the formula above should work just fine. Keep in mind that the amount of protein provided by the formula is more of a maximum than a minimum recommended daily intake. You likely aren't doing yourself any favors by going much above the recommended daily intake so don't feel like you get bonus gains for surpassing it. The recommendation is simply that, a recommendation. Stray a little above or below and it's not a big deal but stray too far in either direction, and you may decrease the operating efficiency of the living machine.

**Amino Acids**

A common misconception about plant-based diets is that plant protein does not provide a complete amino acid profile. Amino acids are what the body breaks protein down into. These compounds are considered the building blocks for life and the body will quite literally wither away without them so if people were missing certain amino acids on a plant-based diet, then that would be pretty concerning. Luckily, every single amino acid that the body needs can be found in all plant foods in varying proportions.[35] These amino acids are in no way inferior from those found in meat.

Another outdated idea that many people still buy into is the need for those on a plant-based diet to meticulously "pair" their proteins to achieve a complete amino acid profile. Since some plants are naturally lower in certain amino acids and higher in others, some people have concluded that you should pair your plant proteins to make up for deficiencies. For example, if beans are low in a certain amino acid and rice is low in a different amino acid, they should be paired together to make up for their respective deficiencies.

This seems like an important idea to consider at face value because of course you don't want to be deficient in any of the nine essential amino acids, the ones your body can't make and must consume. Here's my problem with meticulous plant-based protein pairing: people already do this without thinking about it! Nobody is sitting down and eating a heaping pile of nothing but beans for lunch (at least I hope not). There is really no need to bend over backwards to pair your plant proteins to complete an amino acid profile. If you eat a variety of protein sources, you will be perfectly fine. You don't even have to eat a variety of plant-based protein sources in a single meal to consume a complete amino acid profile. You just need to eat multiple protein sources throughout the day which is incredibly easy to do.

Moreover, once the essential amino acid requirements of the body are met, there is little benefit to consuming additional amino acids. This is because the body will not oxidize these amino acids and use them for muscle protein synthesis since it already has all the amino acids that it needs.[36] What this means is that if you are eating around 20 g of protein in a meal consisting of a variety of different foods, the amino acid profile of these foods really doesn't matter that much. Protein quantity can easily make up for protein quality when it comes to amino acids.

This leads us to another common misconception: that animal protein is somehow superior to plant protein. This is patently false. Protein is protein. We already know that if the proper amount of protein is consumed, the amino acid profile is virtually irrelevant. There is also research showing that if the proper amount of amino acids are consumed, the protein source is irrelevant.[37] If you eat enough protein, not only do you not have to worry about amino acids, the source of this protein also doesn't matter. Put simply, getting your protein from plants instead of animals will in no way impair your quest for gains.

**The Truth About Soy**

Soybeans are one of the top crops currently grown in the U.S. along with wheat and corn. Soy also happens to be a fantastic source of protein for vegans and vegetarians due to its durability, price, and amino acid profile. However, these benefits have put a target on soy's back. Soy fuels a variety of meat replacements like Gardein products and Impossible Foods which cuts directly into the profit of the animal agriculture industry. To combat soy-based meat replacements, the animal agriculture industry has launched a malicious attack on soy products. This attack is typically the false assertion that soy contains estrogen and will therefore make you grow man boobs.

The idea that soy consumption leads to male breasts can be traced back to a highly cited isolated incident back in 2008. Our story begins with a single case study that observed an elderly man suffering from gynecomastia, the enlargement or swelling of male breast tissue. He had an odd habit of consuming three quarts of soymilk a day so his gynecomastia was attributed to this habit since no other explanation could be found.[38] After all, three quarts is a lot of soymilk!

It is important to point out that unlike a peer-reviewed academic journal article, case studies cannot be used to draw conclusions. Typically, as with this case study, the authors end with a question rather than a conclusion. Why can't conclusions be drawn? Because the entire sample studied consisted of a single individual (n = 1). You don't need to be a statistician to see that this is far from the number of subjects needed to perform thorough data analysis, let alone identify a mechanistic cause and effect. Put simply, there are a million reasons why this elderly gentleman could have developed breasts. Despite how it may appear in this singular instance, it is impossible to say that the soymilk was the cause of this man's ailments based on this case study alone. A single case study is insufficient to provide a link between soy and gynecomastia. A single case study is insufficient to find a link between anything for that matter. Case studies serve one purpose: to indicate that further research is needed to explore a topic. So, let's take a look at the research that has investigated the effect of soy on hormones.

A study on Japanese men found that drinking 1.5 cups soymilk/day had no statistical effect on free or total testosterone levels.[39] Another study had young men consume a variety of different protein shakes.[40] They consumed either 50 g of soy concentrate, soy isolate, whey, or a soy isolate/whey blend for 12 weeks. The results demonstrated similar free and total testosterone levels as well as similar lean body mass gains for all groups.

These studies were all performed on younger men, but what about older men like the one in the case study suffering from gynecomastia? A three-month study on men 50 years and up was performed and found that consuming soy in amounts similar to Asian countries (~65 mg isoflavones) had no effect on testosterone.[41] Another 12 week study on men between 50 and 65 that consumed 50 g of soy yogurt (26.7 g protein) daily also found no effect on free testosterone concentrations.[42]

If soy truly has no significant effect on hormones, then certainly a meta-analysis of the entire body of research would indicate this. In 2010, a meta-analysis reviewed 32 different papers and found that the intake of isoflavones, the phytoestrogens found in soy, had no significant effect on testosterone concentrations in men.[43]

It needs to be noted that a handful of conflicting rat studies have observed some impacts on hormones due to phytoestrogen intake. However, these studies had to feed the rats absurd amounts of isoflavones to yield a perceptible signal in the results. Additionally, it's clear that the biology of a rat is a very poor approximation to the biology of a human. One rat study found a 35% reduction in plasma testosterone after consuming 20 mg of isoflavones/kg body weight.[44] If this amount of isoflavones were to be adjusted to the average male human body weight (180 lbs.), it would be the equivalent of approximately 3.5 gallons of soymilk per day! You'd be hard pressed to find a 180 lb. male willing, let alone capable, of consuming such a large quantity of soymilk. I don't think that rat studies like this really carry much weight, especially since they contradict the more robust human studies. In fact, this rat study doesn't even agree with most other rat studies.

A literature review that examined both human and rodent studies concluded that isoflavones do not exert feminizing effects on men at intake levels similar to or even significantly greater than typical Asian males.[45] Historically, Asians have consumed more soy than any other population from products like tofu, soy sauce, miso, tempeh, and edamame yet they are some of the healthiest people in the world. On average, Asians consume roughly 65 mg of isoflavones per day, just 4% of the amount of isoflavones that were fed to the rats in the study mentioned in the previous paragraph.

The animal agriculture industry has pushed the idea that soy will mess with your hormones and possibly make men grow breasts despite the dozens of studies that indicate otherwise. The idea that soy leads to the feminization of men is a myth constructed by the animal agriculture industry to misinform the general public and hurt their plant-based meat competitors.

Soy products do not even contain any real estrogen. Soy only contains phytoestrogen which is incredibly weak. Meat, eggs, and dairy however, all contain real estrogen. If you're concerned about your hormones, what you should really be avoiding are animal products. Hormones are naturally produced in the bodies of all animals so when you consume an animal's flesh, milk, or eggs, you're consuming the animal's hormones along with it.

In addition to the natural hormones in animal products, animals are often injected with synthetic hormones to boost their growth. You consume these too when you eat animal products, especially in dairy. It's difficult to quantify how much estrogen is found in animal products because it varies greatly depending on how the animal was raised and processed. All animal milk contains a relatively high concentration of hormones since biology has designed this liquid to promote infant development. The high concentration of hormones found in dairy products has also been found to be a cancer risk factor of remarkable concern for consumers, producers, and public health authorities.[46] If the animal agriculture industry is really concerned with hormones, they should take a long hard look at their own products before criticizing soy. Instead, they have chosen to push conspiracies with no scientific basis.

As you've likely noticed, all the studies I've mentioned only dealt with men. No, this isn't because I'm sexist. Unfortunately, it's because there's a lack of studies performed on women. Not just soy studies, but medical studies in general typically prefer to work with men because scientists have a better understanding of the male body than the female body. This has everything to do with the fact that historically, men have comprised most of the medical field. It's wrong, it's sexist, but it doesn't change the fact that at this moment I don't have enough scientifically validated research to comment on the effect of female soy consumption on hormones.

However, for men, the research clearly suggests that soy consumption will not lead to any feminizing hormonal changes in humans. In my opinion, if you're not eating meals entirely comprised of soy products or downing gallons of soymilk like there's no tomorrow, then you have absolutely nothing to worry about. I'd argue that men are much more likely to experience feminizing effects from eating animal products, than soy considering that animal foods contain real estrogen. If you're consuming soy phytoestrogen in place of the real estrogen found in animal products, then go enjoy yourself that impossible whopper. Don't allow a myth being spread by the animal agriculture industry to dissuade you from enjoying your food and improving your health.

**Plant-based Protein Sources**

"Where do you get your protein?" This is probably the number one question plant-based athletes get asked. If you decide to adopt a plant-based diet, then be prepared to get this question from nearly everyone who finds out about your diet. Some plant-based folk get frustrated at this question because it's so common. Please stop doing that. If somebody is genuinely curious about your diet, then use this as a teaching opportunity to eradicate the bad assumption that protein only comes from animals. Chances are that if you're like me, at one point you held this bad assumption too. No need to get all woke and take a sincere question personally. With that said, let's get into it.

The short answer to that unavoidable protein question for me is: beans, lentils, nuts, seeds, seitan, tofu, edamame, tempeh, soymilk, whole grains, and protein powder. Along with some indulgence in plant-based meats, which I'll get into later this chapter, this is where I get the bulk of my protein. The answer to the protein question may look different for you though and that's okay. There's a ton of other great plant-based protein sources missing from that list that I didn't include. Nearly all plant foods contain at least some protein, so the options are nearly limitless. Sure, some plant foods are more protein dense than others, but that doesn't mean it's impossible to hit your protein goals by eating none of the foods I have listed above. It all comes down to personal preference at the end of the day.

I prefer to get most of my protein from whole food plant sources to maximize micronutrient intake. This is because these proteins typically come in a superior package in comparison to processed plant protein and especially animal protein. Whole food, plant-based proteins are typically encapsulated in a micronutrient dense package. I consider this packaging as a bonus opportunity to put extra vitamins and minerals into my body to keep it functioning at an optimal level. You miss out on this micronutrient dense package by consuming animal protein in place of plant protein. Some of this package can also be lost by consuming highly processed plant-based protein. During processing, the plant-based protein is often isolated and the micronutrient package surrounding it is discarded.

This doesn't mean you can't have success consuming large quantities of processed meat replacements. I know for a fact that world champion powerlifter, Nick Squires, relies heavily on these products for his protein intake. It just means that if you truly want to optimize the fuel to the living machine, a diet consisting of predominately whole plant foods is probably the way to go. However, meatless meats are still a fantastic addition to your plant-based arsenal in moderation, especially to curb cravings. Nearly every animal product has a plant-based alternative on the market today. Here are a few of my personal favorite plant-based swaps for meals and recipes:

**Beef:**

- Burgers – Beyond Burger, Impossible Burger, Lightlife Plant-Based Burger, Morningstar Farms Meatlovers Vegan Burger
- Hot dogs – Field Roast frankfurter, Lightlife Smart Dogs, Morningstar Farms Veggie Dogs
- Corn dogs – Morningstar Farms Veggie Classics Corn Dogs and Fieldroast Miniature Corndog
- Ground beef – Beyond Beef Plant-Based ground, Beyond Meat Beefy Crumble, Gardein the Ultimate Beefless Ground, Lightlife Ground
- Beef tips – Gardein Beefless Tips and seitan (various brands)
- Meatballs – Lightlife Veggie Meatballs and Gardein Meatless Meatballs

**Chicken:**

- Chicken strips – Quorn Meatless Vegan Filets, Gardein Meatless Chikn Strips, Morning Star Farms Chik'n Strips, and Lightlife Savory Chicken Tenders
- Fried Chicken – KFC Beyond Chicken (currently only at select locations)
- Chicken tenders – Gardein Crispy Tenders and Gardein Nashville Hot Frozen Chik'n Tenders

- Chicken nuggets – Morningstar Farms Veggie Chik'n Nuggets and Boca Original Chik'n Veggie Nuggets
- Popcorn chicken – Morningstar Farms Veggie Classics Popcorn Chik'n
- Chicken patties – Boca Spicy Chik'n Veggie Patty, Boca Original Chik'n Veggie Patty, Morningstar Farms Original Chik Patties, Morningstar Farms Buffalo Chik Patties, and Gardein Crispy Chik'n Patty

**Dairy:**

- Milk – Soymilk, almond milk, cashew milk, oat milk, rice milk, coconut milk, and more. There are more brands than I could possibly list here. Look at the milk section in just about any grocery store and you'll find many of these plant-based milks.
- Butter – Earth Balance, Country Crock Plant Butter, and Smart Balance. All work well as butter spreads and for baking.
- Cheese – Daiya, Go Veggie, Vegan Gourmet, So Delicious, Follow Your Heart, Lisanatti, Good Planet Foods, Violife, and Roast. Between them they have everything from mozzarella, pepperjack, American, cheddar, and parmesan cheese slices, shredded cheese, and sprinkle cheese.
- Ice cream – Breyer's, Ben & Jerry's, Halo Top, Oatly, and So Delicious all have excellent ice cream and between them there's just about every flavor you could dream of. I encourage you to try ice creams made from each plant milk; oat milk, soymilk, almond milk, cashew milk, coconut milk, etc. to figure out which you like best.
- Yogurt – Silk and So Delicious are the easiest ones to find, but there are more brands out there offering vegan yogurt than I could possibly name here. Most of these brands even contain probiotics just like dairy yogurt!
- Ranch – JustRanch and Daiya Homestyle Ranch

**Others:**

- Eggs – Follow Your Heart VeganEgg, JUST Egg, or a good old-fashioned tofu scramble. For baking I recommend making a flax seed egg (ground flax + water), using applesauce, banana, oil, or Bob's Red Mill egg replacer.
- Hot pocket – Gardein Meatless Pepperoni Pizza Pocket
- Pizza rolls – Morningstar Veggitizers Veggie Pepperoni Pizza Bites, Amy's Snacks Vegan Cheese Pizza
- Pork – Gardein Porkless Bites
- Pulled pork – The Jackfruit Company BBQ Jackfruit and Upton's Bar-B-Que Jackfruit
- Turkey – Gardien Lightly Breaded Turk'y Cutlet. This is what I usually eat on thanksgiving and Christmas dinner (it even comes with gravy).
- Sausage – Beyond Sausage, Tofurky Sausage, Field Roast Sausage. Both Field Roast and Beyond Sausage now have breakfast sausages available as well.
- Lunch meat – Tofurky Deli Slices and Lightlife Smart Deli. They have everything from plant-based turkey to ham to bologna currently on the market.
- Pizza – Daiya Dairy-Free Pizza (various topping options) and Amy's Vegan Pizza (various topping options)
- Mac & Cheese – Annie's Vegan Mac, Daiya Dairy-free Deluxe Chedder Style Cheezy Mac, and Field Roast Mac 'n Chao.

Most of these products can be found in just about any grocery store. When in doubt, Whole Foods will likely carry the product you are trying to find. Grocery stores tend to put these items in two locations. The first is a refrigerated section that's usually near the produce and the second is the health foods freezer section. Additionally, some stores also have a section of vegan snacks and non-perishables in the unrefrigerated aisles near other specialty food items. All the products I've listed above are vegan but be aware that vegetarian and non-plant-based organic products often get intermixed with the vegan products at grocery stores so always be sure to check ingredient lists before buying.

**Protein Powder**

A protein powder supplement is highly recommended, especially if you're new to plant-based diets. It's by far the quickest way to get easily absorbable protein into your body after a workout. Most people are familiar with whey protein powder which is derived from dairy byproducts, but there is also a plethora of plant-based protein powders on the market. There are so many plant-based powders out there now that it can be a bit overwhelming. Some of the common plant-based protein supplements include soy, pea, hemp, pumpkin, rice, and wheat. This goes to show that just about anything can be turned into protein powder. With so many plant-based protein powder options how do you go about choosing one?

The best place to start is to analyze the amino acid profile. As previously discussed in the amino acid section of this chapter, it is important to get the full spectrum of amino acids, which are the building blocks of protein. Most people will naturally get all the amino acids they need in a plant-based meal by eating different types of food. The same principle of protein source diversification should be applied to plant-based protein powder by combining different types of powders. This means that the plant-based powders with the best amino acid profile will be blends of multiple types. It seems that a rice/pea protein powder blend is the best way to achieve a balanced amino acid profile. A 60/40 rice/pea blend (60% rice protein by weight and 40% pea protein by weight) has a similar amino acid profile to whey protein powder, the gold standard of protein powders. Let's see how the amino acid profiles compare on the next page for 2 scoops (66 g) of each protein powder:

|                  | **60/40 Rice/Pea Blend** | **Whey** |
|------------------|--------------------------|----------|
| Protein          | 50.9 g                   | 50.1 g   |
| Cystine          | **1.0 g**                | 0.9 g    |
| [E]Histidine     | **1.4 g**                | 1.0 g    |
| [E]Isoleucine    | 2.5 g                    | 2.5 g    |
| [E]Leucine       | **5.1 g**                | 4.8 g    |
| [E]Lysine        | 2.9 g                    | 4.3 g    |
| [E]Methionine    | **1.3 g**                | 0.9 g    |
| [E]Phenylalanine | **3.2 g**                | 1.7 g    |
| [E]Threonine     | 2.2 g                    | **2.5 g**|
| [E]Tryptophan    | 0.6 g                    | **1.0 g**|
| [E]Tyrosine      | **2.9 g**                | 1.3 g    |
| Valine           | **3.0 g**                | 2.5 g    |

*Data obtained from Cronometer

[E]Essential amino acids

    As you can see in the table above, the plant-based protein amino acid profile fairs quite well when compared to whey which is often the go to protein powder for many lifters. Based upon the information in the table above, the amino acid profile of an optimal rice/pea protein blend is superior to that of whey. Seven of the amino acids are more abundant in the plant-based powder, whereas only three amino acids are more abundant in whey. Even when just the essential amino acids are compared, the ones that the body can't produce on its own, the plant-based powder is still superior. The optimized rice/pea blend is more abundant in five of the nine essential amino acids, whereas the whey is more abundant in only three, and they tie on the isoleucine. This is further evidence that those on a plant-based diet probably do not need to stress out about consuming enough of each amino acid. I understand that not every amino acid is listed here, but these are the important ones and the only ones with information available in Cronometer.

    Once the amino acid profile superiority of plant-based protein powder has been revealed, many meat heads may jump to the idea that whey is better because it is more digestible. This is true. Plant-based protein powder tends to be higher in fiber than animal-based protein powders so it can take longer to digest. However, multiple studies comparing whey with plant-based powder found no significant difference between the two protein powders in terms of change in body composition and exercise performance.[47,48] Based upon these studies, it doesn't seem like the digestibility of the protein makes a big difference on the efficacy of the protein powder or at least the difference in digestibility isn't significant enough to be noticeable. A less digestible protein powder isn't necessarily a bad thing anyways. The difference is that less digestible protein powder will just slowly release the protein in your body over time instead of all at once. Some people like this slower burn and seek out slow release protein powders because they report that they are more filling. This is the entire premise behind whey protein powder's cousin, casein, another popular dairy-derived protein supplement.

Even though it doesn't seem to make that big of a difference, maybe you still really want to make sure that your protein powder is digested as quickly as possible. Turns out that when enzymes are added to plant-based powders, the protein powder becomes just as digestible as whey.[49] Enzymes are molecules that help break down food quicker in the body. For those of you that paid attention in chemistry, enzymes are organic catalysts which offer alternative reaction pathways in the body. Digestion is just a chemical reaction, so enzymes offer the living machine an easier way to digest food. The human digestive track already contains numerous enzymes, adding enzymes to protein powder is essentially providing the body with a little digestion boost. Many plant-based powders already have enzymes added to their protein blends. Be on the lookout for this when shopping for protein powder.

I have found the cheapest option for protein powder is to buy pea protein, rice protein, and enzymes in bulk for making my own 60/40 rice/pea protein blend. This may be too much work for some of you. Luckily, there are plenty of good plant-based protein powders out there on the market today. You may have to experiment with a few until you find one that you like. Some dissolve easier than others and some have a chalky texture. The best way around chalky textured protein powders is to blend them into a smoothie. Here's a quick checklist of things to look for when shopping for plant-based protein powders:

**Plant-Based Protein Powder Checklist**

1. Contains both rice and pea protein

2. Reasonably low in carbs and fat (unless you're shopping for weight gain powder)

3. Contains enzymes (only if you're concerned with digestibility)

4. At least 20 g of protein per serving

## Chapter 5: Carbs vs. Fat

An age-old war in the world of nutrition is that between the low-carb and the low-fat dieters. Plant-based diets are typically lumped into the low-fat/high-carb category. Plant-based diets do certainly tend to be high-carb diets, but this is not always the case. There are a lot of athletes out there that consume low-carb/high-fat plant-based diets. One example is plant-based powerlifter and author of *The Vegan Meathead*, Daniel Austin. I highly recommend checking out his book if you're interested in a higher fat plant-based diet. There are also some plant-based folks out there that take their high-fat diet a bit to the extreme, virtually eliminating carbs altogether and consuming vegan keto diets. I personally advise against taking things to this extreme, especially in the long-term, but I see no issue with a moderately high-fat plant-based diet.

Low-carb and low-fat diets are typically designed for weight loss. In 2018, a great study was published that compared the effects of low-fat and low-carb diets on weight loss and there was absolutely no difference in the effectiveness of the two diets.[50] It turns out that there was nothing magical about either of these two diets, they were both just ways to trick people into consuming fewer calories. No matter what the low-carb and low-fat crowds may like you to believe, there really isn't anything special about either of these diets. Do not be fooled into thinking that you are somehow "biohacking" yourself with either of these diets because trust me, there is no outsmarting the living machine. The ketogenic and intermittent fasting diets are both notorious for convincing people that they are somehow cheating the system and entering a magical state of fat burning. Like low-fat and low-carb diets, keto and intermittent fasting are just arbitrary restrictions people can put on themselves to reduce caloric intake. Anybody could come up with a diet that was just as effective at reducing caloric consumption. For example, suppose I invented a diet where you could only eat foods that started with letters A-L. I can almost guarantee this diet would work just as well as any of the other weight loss diets out there. At the end of the day, the only thing that matters for weight loss are calories burned and calories consumed. There is no way around this. Period.

A new ground-breaking study conducted by the National Institute of Health directly compared mostly overweight and obese people on a high-carb vegan diet with those on a low carb animal-based keto diet.[51] This first of its kind study produced some very interesting findings. On average, the vegan group consumed 689 fewer calories than the keto group. Here's where it gets interesting. Despite the lower caloric intake, the vegan group ate 2.1 kg of food on average, whereas the keto group ate 1.4 kg of food on average. The vegans were able to eat more food for fewer calories! Body composition analyses of the patients revealed that the vegan group lost significantly more fat than the keto group and that most of the weight loss in the keto group was from water losses (carbs tend to retain water). If the goal is to lose fat, then it appears that a plant-based diet is superior to that of an animal-based keto diet. However, this doesn't necessarily mean that a low-fat diet is superior to a high-carb diet for weight loss when calories are controlled. It just means that a standard plant-based diet is superior when compared to an animal-based keto diet for weight loss when people are told to eat as much as they want.

If the carb/fat calorie ratio doesn't really matter for weight loss on a plant-based diet, how do you go about selecting macronutrient goals? This answer will be different for everyone and will likely require some trial and error on the part of the reader. It seems to me that some people simply perform better on low-fat diets and others perform better on low-carb diets. In my experience, women typically require a higher proportion of fat than men, this likely has something to do with hormonal differences. Personally, I have tried both low-carb and low-fat plant-based diets and have discovered that a lower-fat (~20% fat) plant-based diet works best for me. This may not be the case for you.

Although the ideal carb/fat ratio does seem to vary from person to person, there is some evidence to suggest that the body benefits from higher carb diets during strength training. One of the main reasons is that carbohydrates are a much more accessible energy source for the body than fat or protein.[52] This means the body could have a harder time fueling itself during an intense lifting session on a low-carb diet. Studies have shown that low-carb diets like keto, atkins, and paleo can increase fatigue and perceived effort during exercise as well as decrease desire to exercise prior to physical activity.[53–55] These effects likely have a lot do with taking away carbohydrates from the body which are its primary source of energy.

Unless you are already certain that low-fat/high-carb diets don't sit well with your body, I recommend upping the carbs when you first go plant-based. Higher-carb plant-based diets probably tend to be a little easier to adhere to considering that most vegan food is higher in carbohydrates. It is also well understood that carbohydrates provide the most accessible source of energy for the body during an intense workout. Finally, if you're not careful, a low-carb/high-fat diet can lead to inflammation if too much saturated fat is consumed.[13] I want to clarify that I'm not advocating for the complete removal of fat or even saturated fat from the diet since the body needs fat to live. However, I do advocate for carbohydrates to be used as your primary source of energy since the living machine has evolved to use carbohydrates as its principal fuel. This can be achieved by ensuring more calories from carbohydrates than fat are consumed.[§] If you give this a shot and don't like it, feel free

---

[§]1 g of carbohydrates contains 4 calories and 1 g of fat contains 9 calories. This means that if you are eating equal grams of fat and carbohydrates, you're getting more than twice as many calories from fat as carbohydrates.

to try a low-carb diet. As previously stated, it doesn't matter all that much to me which approach is chosen. The only thing that matters is that you find the optimal energy source to fuel your body. For lifters, this is more than likely a diet that is higher in carbohydrates. However, the National Academy of Science Food and Nutrition Board's Dietary Reference Intake for fat is 20-35% of your calories so you should probably try to stay within this range.[56] If your daily fat intake drops too far below 20% of your calories, this could potentially be problematic over an extended period of time.

## Chapter 6: Reframing Diet

After learning about protein, fat, and carbs, I think it becomes clear that macronutrients are useful tools, but they shouldn't be the only consideration made when trying to optimize the living machine. Foods shouldn't always be oversimplified and labelled either a protein, carb, or fat. This leaves micronutrients out of the equation and forces people to either demonize or glorify certain macronutrients. Labelling certain nutrients good and other nutrients bad is lazy and counterproductive. The average American has glorified protein and has demonized fat, carbs, and sugar. This has led many overweight Americans astray.

The entire premise of high protein diets being good for weight loss is based upon the idea that high-protein foods are the most satiating form of calories. Contrary to this idea, research has demonstrated that the most satiating foods are not high-protein foods, they are high-fiber foods.[57] This same research found that the most satiating food studied was a potato, not meat. This is because meat and other animal products contain zero fiber. Recall from the previous discussion on the microbiome that the only foods that contain fiber are plant foods. In addition to finding that fiber is more important for satiety than protein, this study also found that fat was one of the least satiating sources of calories. If the goal is to maximize satiety, then the best way to do it is by eating as many whole plant foods as possible and avoiding the consumption of high-fat foods like many animal products. And if maximizing satiety is best way to reduce caloric consumption and promote weight loss, then I'm not convinced that high-protein diets are the best option for those seeking to shed fat.

By glorifying protein, Americans tend consume more calorie dense animal foods like steak, fried chicken, and hamburgers. They view these foods as proteins so therefore, they figure that they can eat as much of these foods as they want. They pay no mind to the fact that excess protein consumption leads to weight gain in the same way excess fat and carbs do or that high fiber plant foods are more satiating than high protein foods. In their blind pursuit to increase protein consumption and lose weight they often inadvertently increase caloric intake. People shouldn't be excluding fiber from their diet in favor of saturated fat and cholesterol. However, this is exactly what many people do. They eat less fruit due to fear of sugar and they eat fewer whole grains and vegetables due to fear of carbs all while increasing the consumption of high-protein animal products. Protein is certainly important, but it isn't everything and you certainly don't have to get it from animals. Think back to the caloric budget. What would be the best way to spend a caloric budget while trying to lose weight? Would you rather eat small portions of calorie dense meat or eat an entire plate of satiating plant foods?

Americans are in desperate need of reframing diet and nutrition. We need to start moving away from the tendency to glorify protein and demonize other nutrients if America is ever going to conquer its obesity epidemic. Due to their satiating high-fiber nature, diets featuring plants appear to be a promising method for reducing obesity. But most plant foods have complex macronutrient profiles so plants can't simply be reduced to a carb, fat, or protein food. This confuses most Americans because they tend to base entire meals around a single source of animal protein. This is demonstrated by the average gym bro meal which is built upon a simple formula:

**Gym Bro Meal = Animal Protein + Carb + Fruit or Vegetable**

For breakfast, the average gym bro will eat eggs with oatmeal and a banana. For lunch, chicken breast with rice and broccoli. For dinner, steak with potatoes and asparagus.

This formula doesn't work all that well when applied to a plant-based diet. A well-designed plant-based diet needs to transcend this gym bro formula to be successful. Instead of applying the conventional approach to nutrition employed by many Americans and viewing foods as either a protein, fat, or carb, I recommend viewing foods as either a fat-based protein, a carb-based protein, a fruit, or a vegetable. The fruits and vegetables are self-explanatory. However, the idea of fat-based proteins and carb-based proteins requires some explanation. Most plant-based sources of protein come along with either a significant amount of carbs or fat. Things like whole grains, beans, and lentils would be considered carb-based proteins, whereas seeds, nuts, and tofu would be considered fat-based proteins. Although I am not a big fan of oversimplifying diet with formulas, I think a simple equation can be provided that is an improvement to the gym bro equation. Here it is:

**Meal = Carb-Based Protein + Fat-Based Protein + Fruit + Vegetable**

This is the simplest meal design I can provide to those who are new to plant-based strength training. This is roughly the template I followed for the first year or so of veganism and it worked well for me. I encourage you to mark this section of the book and return to it later while meal planning. On the next page is a list of recommended foods for you to plug into the above formula:

| Carb-Based Protein | Fat-Based Protein | Fruit | Vegetables |
|---|---|---|---|
| Black beans | Tofu | Apple | Green beans |
| Chickpeas | Pumpkin seeds | Banana | Broccoli |
| Kidney beans | Sunflower seeds | Orange | Carrots |
| Lentils | Avocado | Peach | Brussel sprouts |
| Oatmeal | Peanuts | Blueberries | Asparagus |
| Quinoa | Almonds | Strawberries | Sweet potato |
| Edamame | Cashews | Blackberries | Broccolini |
| Peas | Pistachios | Grapes | Spinach |
| Tempeh | Plant-based meat | Strawberries | Kale |
| Veggie burger | Chia seed | Cherries | Salad |
| Seitan | Peanut butter | Pineapple | Pumpkin |
| Ezekiel bread | Soymilk | Watermelon | Squash |
| Rice | Flax seed | Kiwi | Cabbage |
| Protein pasta | Hemp seed | Mango | Cucumber |
| Millet | Pine nuts | Grapefruit | Celery |
| Buckwheat | Sesame seeds | Plum | Mushrooms |
| Potato | Almond butter | Pear | Peppers |
| Vegan yogurt | Walnuts | Pomegranate | Onion |

Of course, you're welcome to eat foods that are not listed on the above table. I just wanted to provide an easy guide for designing healthy plant-based meals for those who are new to the diet. The idea is to select at least one food from each category to quickly create well-rounded meals rich in protein, quality carbs, healthy fats, and micronutrients. For breakfast I could select potatoes as my carb-based protein, tofu as my fat-based protein, banana as my fruit, peppers as my vegetable and cook up a tofu scramble with the peppers over southern hash browns with a banana on the side. For lunch, I could make a stir fry with rice, edamame, mixed vegetables, and an apple on the side. For dinner, I could make an Italian red sauce protein pasta, with ground beyond beef with a side berry spinach salad. Don't worry about trying to squeeze sauces or condiments into any of the four categories. The formula is just a guideline, not law. It's okay to double up or even triple or quadruple up on some of the categories. Just make sure you try to eat at least one item from each.

# Chapter 7: Supplementation

Supplements are an important part of most high performing athletes' diets. There are some people who have a strong aversion to supplementation because they'd rather stick to a more "natural" approach to diet. Personally, I prefer to use every tool at my disposal in the pursuit of building muscle mass. Regardless of your stance on supplements prior to reading this book, the fact remains that there are supplements necessary for supporting a healthy plant-based diet. These supplements will be discussed in the Essential section of this chapter. Additionally, I have included Recommended and Optional supplement sections. Recommended supplements are those which you should probably be taking to achieve optimal performance, but you should still be able to make decent gains without. Optional supplements are supplements that may or may not lead to direct improvements in performance. The necessity of the optional supplements has more to do with individual differences in physiology and dietary preferences. Most supplements besides those discussed in this chapter are largely snake oil that make egregiously false claims (fat burners, testosterone boosters, etc.) or are supplements that are probably unnecessary for most people.

## Essential Supplements

Vitamin B12

This is the big one. Prior to modern industrialized agriculture, humans used to get all the vitamin B12 they needed with no issue from bacteria. Only bacteria have the ability to synthesize B12.[58] Our ancestors used to be able to easily consume plenty of B12 by simply ingesting small amounts of bacteria loaded dirt from eating unsanitized food and drinking from streams. However, now that industrialized agriculture has become the primary source of food for the developed world, all the B12 producing bacteria is washed away when food and water is sterilized. Don't get me wrong, the increased sanitation of food has saved countless lives so I'm not arguing that this is a bad thing. Humans just need to be cognizant of the fact that we must now supplement vitamin B12.

Even omnivores must consume supplemented vitamin B12. The difference is that they don't have to directly supplement via a pill like those on a plant-based diet. Omnivores get their B12 through consuming animals that consume B12 supplements. No matter how you look at it, everyone must consume supplemented B12 one way or another. It turns out that up to 39% of people, including meat-eaters, are deficient in vitamin B12.[59] This suggests that everyone, not just those on a plant-based diet should probably be directly supplementing B12.

The body has a difficult time absorbing vitamin B12 so don't be alarmed that the back of a bottle of B12 says a single tablet contains 20,000% or more of the daily value of B12. I personally take two 2500 mcg servings of vitamin B12 daily which adds up to over 200,000% of the daily value. Most people would be perfectly fine taking just one of these pills per day, but since I am slightly larger than the average human being, I figure that I might need a little more B12 than most. This might be overkill, but I like to play it safe. The good thing is that it is incredibly difficult to overdose on vitamin B12. Like most vitamins, the body will simply dispose of what it doesn't need via urination.

Don't be fooled into thinking that if you're eating 100% of the daily value of B12 that you're all good and don't need to supplement. The human body absorbs only a small fraction of ingested vitamin B12 so massive doses are needed to get enough of it. I'm a huge fan of nutritional yeast which does contain some B12, but it is nearly impossible to meet the body's B12 requirements through plant foods like this alone. I have seen too many vegans fall into the trap of thinking that they can get all the B12 they need from nutritional yeast or B12 fortified almond milk. That is a risky approach and I strongly advise against it; a much better solution is to take a daily vitamin B12 supplement. Luckily, these vitamins are incredibly inexpensive and can be found in just about any grocery store.

Creatine

Besides vitamin B12, another supplement everyone on a plant-based diet should be taking is creatine monohydrate. This supplement is widely used amongst strength athletes. Like B12, any athlete should probably be taking creatine regardless of whether they consume a plant-based diet. Creatine promotes strength and power output during short-duration, high-intensity workouts, like weightlifting, and has even been shown to increase lean body mass (muscle mass).[60] With these clearly demonstrated benefits, it is no wonder that within the past decade or so creatine has become one of the most popular supplements on the market. It's gotten so popular that some companies even put it in their energy drinks. Those unfamiliar with creatine often fear that it may be unsafe. However, a fairly large body of research has shown that there are no adverse health effects for adults supplementing creatine monohydrate.[61]

The best way to supplement creatine is to take a daily dose with a meal or a protein shake. I recommend purchasing "micronized" creatine monohydrate because it dissolves much easier due to increased surface area. I'll typically add a teaspoon (5 g) of this into my daily post-workout protein shake. Research has shown that moderate daily doses of 3 g per day will saturate the body with creatine within 3-4 weeks.[62] You will find that it is a common theme for me to take just slightly more than the recommended value since I am larger than the average male. Therefore, I take 5 g daily instead of 3 g. Research has also shown that the body may retain supplemented creatine better when it is ingested along with protein and/or carbs.[63] This is why I suggest taking creatine monohydrate during a meal or with a protein shake. If the graininess of the creatine is bothersome, try dissolving the flavorless powder into warm liquid like coffee or tea rather than cool liquid. For those that paid attention in chemistry, solubility is temperature dependent. Warmer doesn't always mean more soluble, but creatine does become much more soluble under warmer conditions.

The body has a certain creatine capacity that it cannot physically exceed no matter how much creatine you supplement. To perform optimally, creatine levels should be maxed out and maintained. For this reason, some people will choose to "cycle" their creatine loading. They will alternate between taking very large doses of creatine and taking little or no creatine. Personally, I see no real benefit to this approach. It doesn't seem like a good idea to periodically deplete the body's creatine storage like this just to turn around and max it out again. I would much rather max out the body's creatine storage capacity and maintain it at its peak by taking daily moderate doses.

There are a few potential negative side effects to keep in mind with creatine supplementation. Mild gastrointestinal distress has been reported by some and I have personally experienced this when I tried upping my daily creatine intake to 15 g per day at one point.[64] Any potential digestive issues usually subside after a week or two. If this side effect is particularly unbearable, I would suggest slowly ramping up daily creatine intake. Another thing to keep in mind when supplementing creatine is that it can increase water retention. Creatine will cause the body to draw water into the muscle so there may be some water-induced weight gain as a result. Since more water is going to the muscle, it is a good idea to drink extra water throughout the day to avoid becoming dehydrated. All in all, these are small potential prices to pay for the nearly certain benefits that creatine supplementation can yield. If you're not already using creatine, I suggest you go out and buy in bulk because it's about to become your new best friend.

**Recommended**

Protein Powder

I've already covered a lot of the details surrounding plant-based protein powders in the Chapter 4. I showed you how a good rice/pea blend can be just as, if not more, effective than whey protein powder. It's possible to get jacked without ever touching protein powder, but a drinkable protein supplement is incredibly convenient. This is especially true if you have trouble eating enough throughout the day. It doesn't get much easier than slapping some powder into a blender bottle and gulping down 20+ g of protein. I highly recommend at least incorporating a post-workout protein shake into your diet, especially if you are unable to eat a solid post-workout meal immediately after your training sessions.

Probiotic

Probiotics are live bacteria that aid the digestion process in the human gut. In addition to eating plenty of prebiotic fiber, gut health can also be promoted by taking a probiotic supplement. The bacteria in the gut feeds on dietary fiber. Therefore, the best way to optimize gut health is to consume lots of fiber and regularly introduce new helpful bacteria to the gut microbiome. Remember, a healthy microbiome is a big edge because it allows the body to absorb micronutrients more efficiently. Not only that, but healthy intestinal bacteria will even manufacture their own micronutrients like vitamin K and some B vitamins.[65] Large quantities of probiotics can be consumed in plant-based foods like miso, tempeh, and many vegan yogurts, but can also be more conveniently supplemented in a daily pill capsule. A probiotic supplement essentially supercharges the already healthy plant-based gut microbiome by introducing it to new kinds of bacteria that it may be lacking.

There is also a lot of evidence showing that gut bacteria may also play a role in preventing obesity and helping keep the body lean.[66] Researchers have recently been exploring potential relationships between gut bacteria and hormones. There is emerging research suggesting that gut bacteria could be communicating with the brain trough hormones and influencing appetite.[67] This would help explain how a healthy microbiome can prevent you from overeating and becoming obese. Perhaps you may not be in danger of becoming obese, but I'm sure we could all benefit from a little more appetite control, especially if your goal is to get lean and mean.

When shopping for probiotics I would shop for something that contains at least 25 billion CFU which stands for colony-forming unit. CFU is a measure of the number of bacteria per serving. The higher the CFU, the more potent the probiotic. Another thing to look out for when shopping around for probiotics is that the supplement should contain a wide variety of different types of bacteria in it. There are many strains of gut bacteria, so it is important to be introducing a diverse population of various strains when supplementing. The strain types will usually be listed in italics on the back of the bottle (they're the long Latin names). When it comes to strains of bacteria in probiotics, the more the merrier. Since every probiotic supplement is different, you should periodically change which brand of probiotic supplement you use to ensure that you are introducing a diverse range of bacteria to the gut.

Vitamin D

Believe it or not, the best source of vitamin D is not dietary, it comes from the sun. When ultraviolet rays from the sun hit your skin, it provides the energy to kickoff vitamin D synthesis. Therefore, getting all the vitamin D you need in the winter or in regions where there is less sun is difficult. Since the body can produce vitamin D, it is technically not a vitamin. It is a hormone precursor, also referred to as a prohormone.

The human body requires this prohormone, more commonly referred to as vitamin D, to absorb calcium and promote bone growth. Like most vitamins, it also supports a wide variety of roles in the body including immune function and cardiovascular health. Additionally, vitamin D can reduce inflammation and enhance neuromuscular function which is beneficial to exercise performance. Unfortunately, about 42% of all Americans are vitamin D deficient so there is a good chance you may be amongst them.[68] The easiest way to prevent a vitamin D deficiency is to take a daily supplement. The recommended daily intake of Vitamin D for most adults is 600 IU (15 mcg) so look for a supplement that will help you meet this recommendation.[69] It can be difficult to find a vegan vitamin D supplement at the grocery store so I suggest looking online.**

## BCCA's

Branch-chained amino acids (BCAAs) consist of three amino acids: leucine, isoleucine, and valine. The BCAAs represent about 35-40% of all essential amino acids in the body, 15-18% of which are found in the body's muscles.[70] These three amino acids are particularly valuable to muscle recovery, especially leucine which acts as a foreman and tells the body to start building new muscle mass.[71] BCAAs have been used for quite a while by elite athletes. Not only because they taste great, but because there is a growing body of research that champions their efficacy. Some research has shown that consuming BCAAs during exercise helps reduce fatigue.[72] For this reason, I'd

---

**When shopping for supplements, always be sure to read the ingredients. Pill capsules will often be composed of gelatin which is an animal product derived from the skin, tendons, ligaments, and bones of cows and pigs. Fortunately, many of the places you purchase supplements will sometimes have versions of the supplements that do not come wrapped in animal products. It's also very easy to find vegan supplements online.

recommend using BCAAs as an intra workout supplement rather than a pre or post workout supplement. Additionally, there is a significant amount of research showing that the consumption of BCAAs can reduce the dreaded delayed onset muscle soreness (DOMS) by up to 33%.[73–75] Reducing DOMS is critical to speeding up recovery so that you can get back into the gym to make more gains as soon as possible. BCAAs are also often prescribed to those suffering from a critical illness like cancer to help prevent muscle degradation, but research on how effectively it accomplishes this is limited.[76]

It is possible to get all the BCAAs you need through food alone on a plant-based diet. Nevertheless, BCAA supplements are great if you think there is a chance that you may not be consuming enough leucine, isoleucine, or valine throughout the day. An easy way to check this is to track all your food for a day in the Cronometer app and look at the detailed report under the protein section. Overall, BCAAs are not necessary for fueling the living machine, but they are recommended.

Omega-3 Fatty Acids

Omega-3's are polyunsaturated fatty acids that play a variety of important roles in the human body. Research has shown that omega-3's improve just about everything from mental disorders to bone and joint health.[77,78] As more research is conducted, the list seems to keep growing. An omega-3 is considered an essential fatty acid because humans are incapable of synthesizing this compound themselves so they must consume this nutrient. There are three types of omega-3's: α-linolenic acid (ALA), eicosapentaenoic acid (EPA), and docosahexaenoic acid (DHA). ALA is found in plant oils, whereas EPA and DHA are found in marine oils.

A few years ago, fish oil became a trendy supplement and everyone including myself was popping one daily (back before I was plant-based). Few really understood why, we just thought it was the healthy thing to do and knew it had something to do with omega-3's. Health magazines seemed to have convinced everyone that we were all deficient in omega-3's. It turns out that what had really happened was that doctors realized that the ratio of omega-6's, another fatty acid, to omega-3's was too high. The recommended ratio of omega-6 to omega-3 fatty acids is 4:1. However, the standard American diet, or SAD as I like to call it, often consists of a ratio as high as 50:1. The reason behind this is that most SAD people were simply eating too much omega-6 in their greasy westernized diets. These people aren't necessarily omega-3 deprived, they were just eating way too much omega-6.

The fish oil industry really took off from omega-3 deficiency fear mongering, but the only reason fish are rich in omega-3's is that they consume algae and phytoplankton. As with many vital nutrients, it turns out that plants are the original source of omega-3's. This is good news because it means that there are plenty of vegan omega-3 supplements out there that have extracted the nutrient from marine plants and put it into a convenient pill form. Unfortunately, as the world's waters become more polluted, vegans and omnivores alike may want to start using plant-based omega-3 supplements rather than fish oil. Fish bioaccumulate many toxins in their bodies such as mercury and unfortunately, oils are especially good at absorbing these toxins.[79] This means that some of the nasty chemicals that humans dump into bodies of water are ending up in fish oil pills.

If your diet contains at least a moderate amount of fat and you consume omega-3-rich plant foods like flax seed and chia seed regularly, you may not need to supplement. To figure out if you do need to supplement, I once again would recommend downloading the Cronometer app and tracking an average day of eating. The app will display your omega-3 intake in the daily report under the fat section. If your omega-3 intake is too low, then it's probably time to start looking for a supplement or time to incorporate more flax and chia seed into your diet. When searching for a vegan omega-3 supplement, be sure it includes both EPA and DHA. You shouldn't need to worry about ALA on a diet with a moderate amount of fat because it is easy to consume enough from everyday foods since plant oils are rich in ALA.

## Zinc

Zinc is an essential micronutrient that is the second most abundant trace metal in the human body.[80] This is an indication that the body relies upon zinc for a wide variety of functions. Zinc has been shown to promote immune function, heart health, and reduce inflammation.[81-83] As is the case with most micronutrients, it is possible for those on a completely plant-based diet to consume all the zinc that they need through diet alone. Plant foods such as nuts, seeds, and legumes are all rich in zinc. Those who consume a predominately whole foods diet likely eat plenty of these zinc-rich plants, but those who rely heavily upon processed plant foods likely eat fewer of these zinc-rich foods making them more susceptible to a zinc deficiency. Because of this, some research has shown that vegetarians tend to consume slightly less zinc than non-vegetarians.[84] This doesn't necessarily mean that you are doomed to become zinc deficient on a plant-based diet, you just need to pay a little extra attention to your zinc consumption. If you don't consume enough zinc with an average day of eating, then it's time to start taking a daily zinc supplement or incorporating more zinc-rich foods into your diet. Once again, I suggest using Cronometer to monitor zinc intake.

## **Optional**

### Glucosamine, Chondroitin and MSM

These three supplements are often packaged together in the same pill because they are all used to treat joint issues. Once you start moving some serious poundage in the gym, your joints will likely take a beating. It's important to keep an eye out for your joint health to prevent injury, especially if you're older. Glucosamine and chondroitin are used in the body to develop and maintain the cartilage in your joints. Some research has indicated that methylsulfonylmethane (MSM) may enhance the effectiveness of glucosamine and chondriotin.[85,86]

With that said, the evidence that these joint supplements are 100% effective is a little shaky. There are a lot of conflicting studies when it comes to these supplements. A 2010 meta-analysis showed no difference between a glucosamine/chondroitin pill and a placebo for treating hip and knee joint pain.[87] However, some studies do report promising results demonstrating these supplements may help reduce inflammation and cartilage degradation.[88,89] If the evidence was clearer that these supplements worked, they would probably be bumped up from being optional to being recommended. I have personally been taking this supplement for many years in hopes of mitigating joint pain, but until more studies are conducted, it is unclear how well they are working. If you do decide to take one of these joint supplements, be sure to check the ingredients because I've been fooled into buying joint supplements that contain shellfish before. There are vegan versions of this supplement out there, but you will likely have to order them online.

Magnesium

Nearly half of the U.S. population fails to meet recommended magnesium intakes.[90] This is problematic because magnesium is vital for human health. It is an especially critical nutrient for lifters because magnesium helps enhance muscle performance and recovery.[91] Greens, nuts, seeds, and whole grains are all good plant-based sources of magnesium, but some people may need to supplement. Monitor a day of eating with Cronometer to figure out whether you should be taking a magnesium supplement. One thing to keep in mind if you do decide to supplement magnesium is that this is definitely not a pre workout supplement. Magnesium tends to induce drowsiness, so I usually take a high dose each night right before going to bed. Another thing to keep in mind is that calcium, magnesium, and zinc all compete for absorption in your body so avoid buying calcium/magnesium/zinc supplements. It is best to spread out or "stack" each of these metals as much as possible to optimize absorption. Otherwise, you're just making some really nutrient dense urine.

Beta-alanine

Beta-alanine is an important amino acid, but it is non-essential, meaning that your body can synthesize this amino acid itself. Beta-alanine helps the body produce a chemical called carnosine. This carnosine is stored in skeletal muscle and helps reduce the accumulation of lactic acid in the muscles during exercise and this lack of lactic acid accumulation promotes exercise performance.[92] This raises the question of "why not just take carnosine supplements directly instead of taking beta-alanine to indirectly raise carnosine levels?" Research has shown that a beta-alanine supplement does a better job at raising carnosine levels than directly taking carnosine.[93]

Although research strongly suggests that beta-alanine supplements are beneficial, there are some minor side effects. If you've ever felt tingly after taking pre-workout, this is due to beta-alanine. Don't worry, despite the weird side effect, the International Society of Sports Nutrition has found that beta-alanine is a perfectly safe supplement.[94] However, I recommend starting out with smaller doses to see how your body reacts to the supplement. I've taken too much on a handful of occasions and have had to postpone workouts due to overwhelming tinginess that sometimes leads to nausea. The recommended daily dosage is 2-5 g so either start out on the lower end or space out dosages.[95] Beta-alanine is a flavorless soluble powder so it's easy to mix into a preworkout drink or a smoothie. The timing of beta-alanine supplementation doesn't seem to matter very much so just take it daily when convenient.

Caffeine and Pre-workout

I'm sure everyone is already well-acquainted with this supplement and most use it regularly, but I consider it optional.

Caffeine is the primary active ingredient found in pre-workout so I've lumped these two supplements together. However, things like beta-alanine, BCAAs, and creatine can also often be found in pre-workout, but I've already covered these in depth.

Personally, I am not the biggest fan of caffeine and pre-workout. Caffeine makes me feel jittery and I develop caffeine reliance very quickly which gives me headaches. If you're anything like me, you're probably better off without caffeine. If you like caffeine and pre-workout, then that's great. Though, don't feel like you NEED to be taking pre-workout to get jacked because that's simply not true. Coffee gets the job done just as well if you need to get hyped up before a lifting session. I personally find that relying on caffeine to get a good lift can be problematic in the long-term. Eventually, the body gets used to the caffeine intake and requires larger doses to yield the same effect you were getting before. This inevitably leads to either an ever-increasing intake of caffeine or a decrease in performance. Neither of these outcomes seem particularly appealing to me. Because of this, I only use caffeine as a last resort to get me through a lift.

Leucine

Leucine is one of the essential amino acids that the body cannot produce on its own. It is the most important ingredient in BCAAs due to its large role in muscle protein synthesis. Because it is so important, some may people may choose to supplement leucine on its own without the other amino acids. The benefit of doing this is that the leucine doesn't have to compete to be absorbed by the body with isoleucine and valine, the other two BCAAs. Some research has shown that the ingestion of leucine along with protein may promote muscle protein synthesis more than just the ingestion of protein alone.[37,96,97] The research surrounding leucine supplementation is still emerging, but it is clear that leucine plays a critical role in building new muscle.

Something I have been trying out recently is to take a leucine supplement 15-30 minutes before drinking a protein shake. Since leucine essentially tells the other amino acids to start building muscle, the idea is to spike the leucine levels in my blood prior to consuming the protein. This way, by the time the protein enters my body, the leucine concentration is peaking in the blood and the leucine can immediately direct the body to start using the protein to build new muscle. If I were to take the leucine with my protein shake or a meal, the carbohydrates in these protein sources may slow down the leucine absorption and my blood leucine levels wouldn't be primed before the protein arrived.[98] This approach is based on reasonably limited information so until more research can confirm my speculations, leucine supplementation will remain in the optional section.

Iron

Iron is the most abundant trace metal in the human body with most of that iron being in the blood. Plant-based diets are often criticized for being low in iron, but recent studies have shown that vegan and vegetarian diets contain just as much, if not more iron than omnivorous diets.[99–101] This is because whole plant foods like nuts, seeds, legumes, whole grains, and vegetables are great sources of iron. However, as previously discussed, the nonheme iron found in plants is less bioavailable than the heme iron found in animals. This isn't necessarily a bad thing since animal sourced heme iron is absorbed so quickly by the body that it leads to inflammation which can slow muscle recovery.[11] So if you can consume enough nonheme iron throughout the day from plant sources, you are probably better off than if you were consuming the more bioavailable, but inflammatory, heme iron. The American Dietetic Association recommends that those on plant-based diets strive for 1.8 times the recommended daily iron intake just to be safe.[99] This equates to a daily intake of 10.8 mg of iron for adult men and a higher intake of 14.6 mg for adult women due to menstrual losses.[102] Hitting these targets is much easier than it sounds because so many plant foods are rich in iron. I regularly consume 80+ mg of iron, about 7.5 times the recommended daily iron intake, so chances are you'll hit your iron target without even trying.

As easy as these iron targets are to hit, about 5.6% of Americans suffer from anemia which is primarily caused by iron deficiency and can lead to a wide variety of poor health outcomes.[103] If you suffer from anemia or regularly fail to meet the recommended daily intake of iron, then an iron supplement is something to strongly consider. Additionally, research has shown that consuming vitamin C with iron can increase absorption by up to 67%.[104] Considering vitamin C is almost exclusively found in plant foods, it is not surprising that most people on a plant-based diet don't have much to worry about when it comes to iron deficiency in comparison to meat-eaters. Additionally, there has been some limited research suggesting that dairy consumption may increase the risk of iron deficiency.[105] This is something to keep in mind, especially for vegetarians who heavily rely upon dairy products. Anecdotally, I have heard of a handful of cases of vegetarians overcoming iron deficiency by transitioning to veganism and removing dairy from their diet. More research needs to be conducted on this, but it is something to consider.

Calcium

It is common knowledge that calcium helps build strong bones, but not so common knowledge that dairy is far from the best source of calcium. Dark leafy green vegetables, tofu, and soymilk are all much better sources of this nutrient. The average human requires about 1,000-1,200 mg of calcium per day. If you consume a well-rounded plant-based diet, you shouldn't have much trouble with this. One of the most obvious side effects of a calcium deficiency is an increase in bone fractures. People often argue that vegans and vegetarians are more susceptible to bone fractures due to potential calcium deficiency. However, there is conflicting research on whether those on a plant-based diet suffer from more bone fractures than omnivores.[106-108] It's difficult to draw conclusions from these conflicting studies, but this would indicate that calcium is something that everyone should probably pay attention to.

Before you run out and buy a calcium supplement, there is some critical information that needs consideration. Some research has shown that it may be harmful to consume more than the recommended 1,000-1,2000 mg calcium intake because it can lead to decreased iron and zinc absorption as well as potentially harmful calcium build up in soft tissue.[69] If this was not the case, then calcium may have been promoted from an optional to a recommended supplement. However, based on the existence of negative side effects from overconsuming calcium, a calcium supplement should probably only be taken to make up for a deficiency. Tracking your food in the Cronometer app is a great way to identify potential calcium deficiencies.

Superfood Powder and/or Multivitamin

Superfood powder and multivitamin supplements have been lumped into the same category because they both serve the same purpose. They provide a variety of different vitamins and minerals to the body in moderate amounts all at once. The main difference between superfood powder and a multivitamin is that one is in powder form and the other is in pill form. Both supplements are popular amongst the general population, but I don't think either are necessary. The primary purpose they serve would be to make up for any nutritional deficiencies in your diet that you may have missed. The problem is that by introducing all these vitamins and minerals into the body at once, your body only absorbs a small fraction of them. Spreading out various individual vitamins and minerals throughout the day is a better approach to maximize absorption.

Overall, I would not recommend taking one of these supplements to make up for a deficiency. For example, if you are deficient in zinc, then you should be taking a daily zinc supplement not a multivitamin or superfood powder.

Multivitamins and superfood powders are convenient options for people who are unaware of their nutritional intakes. However, if you want to make gains then you should strive to have a nutritional awareness. This has never been easier to do with food tracking apps like Cronometer or MyFitnessPal. I would urge you to use these apps to identify any nutritional deficiencies and treat them with the respective individual supplements rather than slapping a multivitamin or superfood band-aid on the deficiency. Once you develop an awareness of your average nutritional intake and want to use one of these supplements to get an extra dose of micronutrients then go for it. I personally use a superfood powder in my daily smoothies for this purpose.

# Chapter 8: Plant-Based Strength Masters

There is much to be learned from the pioneers in vegan strength sports. The four athletes you will soon become acquainted with are exceptional competitors in their respective sport of choice. Plant-based diet aside, these athletes have reached heights on the world stage that few have before. Fueled by plants, they have become the elite of the elite and regardless of whether you wish to compete or not, there is a thing or two to be learned from these athletes. Each athlete has taken a different approach to their plant-based diet. By studying and interacting with them, I hope to share the wisdom that these plant-based strength masters have acquired. Pay close enough attention and perhaps you may have the opportunity to walk amongst the vegan gods someday as a plant powered champion.

## Patrik Baboumian: *Germany's Strongest Man*

Prior to adopting a plant-based diet, Patrik shattered my perception that vegans are frail and weak. This brutish man resembles a mixture of wolverine and the hulk. After a successful amateur bodybuilding career, he adopted a vegetarian diet in 2005 and went on to win Germany's Strongest Man in 2011. Patrick made waves in the media when shortly after being crowned as Germany's Strongest Man, he announced that he would be upping the ante on his plant-based diet by going vegan. The critics said his muscles would shrivel, but after adopting a vegan diet, he went on to break multiple strongman world records in the beer keg lift, front hold, log lift, and yoke walk. He even briefly changed gears to powerlifting and became the European Raw Powerlifting Champion in 2012. In terms of strength sports, this guy has excelled at it all.

It's difficult to understate the importance of Patrik's success for promoting plant-based diets. He was truly a plant-based strongman pioneer. He dared to diverge from the worn path left behind by the strongman before him. A strongman diet is typically characterized by massive amounts of animal products, but Patrik came along and demonstrated that this was unnecessary to build the mass needed to be a successful strongman. This changed the world of strength sports forever. Even World's Strongest Man, Hafþor Björnsson, aka The Mountain, who recently set a controversial world deadlift record of 501 kg (1,104 lbs.), has now indicated that he would be open to giving veganism a shot.[109] It's hard to imagine that The Mountain, a previously self-proclaimed "carnivore" would have been open to a plant-based diet prior to Patrik's success.

In the world of strongman, competitors must consume enormous amounts of calories to build the mass needed for competition. This could pose a challenge for plant-based lifters since most foods in plant-based diets tend to have a large volume to calorie ratio. Patrik has managed to overcome this challenge by utilizing easily digestible liquid calories. He has outlined what a typical day of eating looks like for him on his YouTube channel.[110] Although he admits that his diet changes frequently, a template of his diet that he has provided is shown below:

**Patrik Baboumian Meal Plan**

**5,320 calories, 410 g protein, 470 g carbs, 200 g fat**

| Meal | Description |
| --- | --- |
| Pre-Workout Meal | Protein shake with creatine and beta alanine |
| Post-Workout Meal | Protein smoothie* |
| Lunch | Vegan sausage, falafel, baked fries, and peppers |
| Snack 1 | Protein shake with omega-3 oil |
| Dinner | Tofu, zucchini with curry paste, peppers, and boiled potatoes |
| Snack 2 | Peanuts |
| Snack 3 | Protein shake |

*Recipe found in Chapter 9

**Nimai Delgado:** *IFBB Pro Bodybuilder*

This lifelong vegetarian and fellow engineer rose the ranks in bodybuilding shortly after going vegan in 2015. The following year, Nimai became the NPC National Champion in Men's Physique. This earned him his IFBB pro card allowing him to be recognized as a professional bodybuilder internationally. Nimai shocked the world with his ability to develop a chiseled aesthetic on a plant-based diet, but this was of little surprise to other plant-based athletes who have experienced the power of plants firsthand. In fact, as far back as the 50s and 60s, Bill Pearl set the stage for plant-based bodybuilders as a vegetarian Mr. Universe. Nimai provided further evidence of the power of plants by never consuming meat since the time he was born and by launching a successful bodybuilding career on an entirely plant-based vegan diet.

Nimai bases his diet around high protein whole plant foods which are conducive to building lean muscle. While Niami's competitors consumed chicken breast and egg whites day in and day out, he ate a more diversified diet built around tempeh, lentils, nuts, edamame, tofu, seeds, hemp, beans, quinoa, rice, hummus, oatmeal, and potatoes. The biggest benefit for plant-based bodybuilders is that they can consume more volume while cutting than their omnivorous peers. Whole plant foods are packed with fiber and micronutrients that won't lead to weight gain the way calorie dense meats will when eaten in the same volume. This meant that leading up to competition, Nimai could still eat large plates of food while other bodybuilders were nibbling on small portions of chicken breast and a few spears of asparagus. Here's what a typical day of eating looks like for Nimai:

**Nimai Delgado Meal Plan**

| Meal | Description |
| --- | --- |
| Breakfast | Protein shake |
| Lunch | Tempeh, tofurky sausage, sweet potato, and cabbage |
| Pre-Workout Meal | High calorie protein shake: protein powder, oatmeal, sunflower butter, flax seed, and dates |
| Post-Workout Meal | Rice, quinoa, curry, sweet potato, chutney |
| Dinner | Tempeh, mixed vegetables, 2 sweet potatoes |

**Nick Squires:** *IPL World Champion Powerlifter*

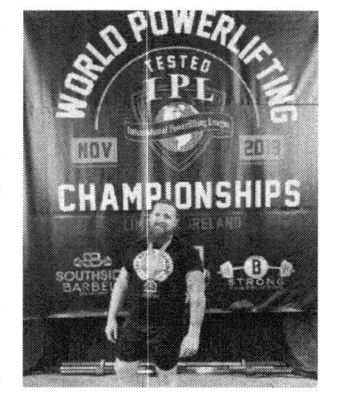

In 2019, Nick Squires became the first vegan to capture an International Powerlifting League World Championship. In the 231 lb. weight class, this beast of a man deadlifted a massive 666.9 lbs. that propelled him to a 1603.8 lb. raw total to secure his spot as a world champion. This performance was also achieved in a drug-tested powerlifting league, so anybody looking to credit steroids to his success as a plant-based athlete should sit down. More recently, Nick has dropped down to the 220 lbs. weight class where he currently holds the California state record in the deadlift.

Nick is obviously a force to be reckoned with, so how does this massive man fuel his training? He is an avid proponent of the wide variety of meat replacements out on the market today. On any given day, you can catch Nick chowing down on a vegan burger after a big squat session or demolishing some vegan doughnuts after pulling 585 for reps.

According to Nick, "Before going vegan, I ate fast food three meals a day, and what drew me to veganism was that I could stop eating animals without having to give up the foods I loved. I do eat significantly better now with a much better balance of fruits and vegetables, but cheeseburgers still play a large role in my diet. Powerlifting demands a lot of protein and calories, and the foods I enjoy happen to provide them, so it's a win-win."

His approach to nutrition is like that taken by most of the powerlifting community: eat whatever allows you to consume as many calories as possible as easily as possible. Like most powerlifters, Nick says, "My biggest concerns as a powerlifter are calories and protein, so I look for things that are high in both." The key point of divergence in Nick's approach compared to most powerlifters is that these calories are sourced exclusively from plants. See what an average day of eating looks like for Nick on the next page:

**Nick Squires' Bulking Meal Plan**

**5,000 calories, 250 g protein**

| Meal | Description |
| --- | --- |
| Breakfast | Tofu scramble w/ onions, bell peppers, spinach, and buffalo sauce |
| Snack 1 | Clif Builders Bar |
| Lunch | Morning Star Chick'n chana masala |
| Snack 2 | PB&J |
| Dinner | Pasta with a plant-based beef sauce or Gardein "meatballs" |
| Snack 3 | Lenny & Larry's Complete Cookie |

Nick has achieved high levels of athletic performance by adapting the powerlifting community's standard approach to nutrition to fit a plant-based diet. There is beauty in the simple nature of Nick's diet. Consuming what many would consider to be "processed junk" is incredibly efficient for a powerlifter. This food typically digests quickly and doesn't fill you up which seems like a negative to most but is advantageous for a powerlifter that requires a massive caloric intake. Not too many people out there could manage to consume 5,000+ calories exclusively sourced from whole plant foods. The amount of fiber alone that would come along with such a diet would bloat any normal human into a balloon and render them incapable of training.

There are also big advantages to taking Nick's simple approach to diet for those just beginning their plant-based journey. First and foremost, it allows beginners to continue to eat the foods they enjoy and curb their cravings. Craving pizza? Eat a vegan pizza. Craving ice cream? Go get some vegan ice cream. This approach is incredibly beneficial to diet adherence because at the end of the day, nothing is truly being given up. Foods containing animal products are simply replaced with versions that are animal product-free, and typically healthier. It's a win-win.

Although Nick's diet may not be ideal for a bodybuilder who often meticulously selects their source of calories, it has a variety of benefits for those seeking to build raw strength. The approach can be gloriously summarized as: eat a lot of high protein plant food that tastes good. So simple it's stupid.

**Kendrick Farris:** *American Olympic Weightlifter*

Kendrick Farris made headlines when he became the only Team USA male weightlifter to qualify for the 2016 Rio Olympics. Fueled by his vegan diet, Kendrick broke the U.S. record during the Olympic trials with a total of 831 lbs. by lifting 370 lbs. in the snatch and 461 lbs. in the clean and jerk. He claims that his vegan diet has significantly improved his recovery speed and focus which helped him achieve this great feat.

Prior to going vegan in 2014, Farris was obsessed with tracking everything he put into his mouth. Farris now refuses to apply any strict limitations to his diet. He simply eats when hungry, shoots for a wide range of different plant foods in his diet, and eats what makes him feel strong during training. After all, getting too caught up in restrictions can take away from how fun training on a plant-based can be. Farris doesn't claim to have any go-to supplements, only using them occasionally to supplement his vegan diet. A sample of what Kendrick Farris eats in a day can be seen below:

**Kendrick Farris Meal Plan**

| Meal | Description |
| --- | --- |
| Breakfast | Pancakes and fresh fruit (usually grapefruit or berries) |
| Snack | Protein shake and trail mix |
| Lunch | Spinach lasagna |
| Post-workout Meal | Black bean chips and guacamole |
| Dinner | Black bean quesadillas |

Farris relies upon an intuitive approach to his nutrition and eats throughout the day rather than consuming two or three large tracked meals. I'd imagine a plant-based strength master probably has a good intuition when it comes to their dietary needs. Many of them are capable of visually assessing their plate and determining what they need to eat to fuel their training. I have used this approach from time to time, but it is an acquired skill. Certainly, not something that beginners to plant-based diets should rely upon. However, I do think achieving balance is important. Lifting on a plant-based diet should be fun and being too meticulous with tracking your food shouldn't take away from that.

**Honorable Mentions**

- Alison Crowdus: *Powerlifter, National Bench Press Record-holder*
- Andreas Cahling: *IFBB Pro Bodybuilder, Mr. International*
- Barny du Plessis: *Bodybuilder, Amateur Mr. Universe*
- Bill McArthy: *Powerlifter, 3x USAPL American Open Champion*
- Bill Pearl: *IFBB Pro Bodybuilder, 5x Mr. Universe*
- Clarence Kennedy: *Olympic Weightlifter and Powerlifter*
- Crissi Carvalho: *IFBB Pro Bodybuilder*
- Hulda B. Waage: *Powerlifter, Iceland National Bench and Squat Record-holder*
- Ilya Ilyin: *Olympic Weightlifter, 2x Gold Medalist*
- Jehina Malik: *IFBB Pro Bodybuilder*
- Jim Morris: *IFBB Pro Bodybuilder, Masters Olympia Champion*
- Karl Bruder: *World Amateur Bodybuilding Association Champion*
- Kim Best: *Strongwoman, Scotland's Strongest Woman Runner-up*
- Natalie Matthews: *IFBB Pro Bodybuilder*
- Torre Washington: *IFBB Pro Bodybuilder*
- Varinder Ghuman: *IFBB Pro Bodybuilder, Mr. India, and Mr. Asia Runner-up*

## Chapter 9: Recipes

Going fully plant-based has granted me the opportunity to explore spices and foods I never would've encountered otherwise. I have taken full advantage of the abundance of plants out there and have tried new foods often. Most Americans consume the same five animals their entire life: cows, pigs, chickens, fish, and turkeys. There are hundreds of thousands of plants out there that these people are missing out on because they're too busy filling up their caloric budget with bland eggs, milk, and flesh. When you think about it, the only thing that make most animal products palatable are plants! People will cover their animal products in plant-based spices and sauces to enhance their flavor instead of just eating the plants. Have you ever tried unseasoned boiled chicken breast? It's difficult to imagine anything blander than that. However, when you add some plants to it, then it suddenly becomes edible.

I strongly advise that when you begin your plant-based journey to not avoid foods that appear exotic or unusual in the context of a standard American diet. If you simply take an American diet and remove the animal products from it, you will be missing out on all that a plant-based diet has to offer. Turn to Middle Eastern, Thai, Japanese, Mexican, Chinese, Indian, Jamaican, and Ethiopian food for starters if you need some culinary inspiration. Each of these unique cultures offer delicious dishes that are completely animal product free. I encourage you to try your hand at cooking a couple of authentic dishes from these cultures using quality fresh ingredients. You will walk away from the experience with an enhanced palate and cooking knowledge essential to your strength journey.

Believe it or not, being a good cook can significantly enhance your ability to adhere to a healthy diet. It is much easier to eat healthy when the food tastes good. If you can figure out how to make a micronutrient dense meal just as delicious as your favorite less healthy meals, then you are on your way to swole city. I know many of you may not have time to go grocery shopping and cook every meal you consume and that's okay. As a PhD student, I understand the constraints associated with time limitations. Personally, I find it easiest to simply dedicate Saturday mornings to grocery shopping and then dedicate Sundays to meal prepping. On Sundays, I will prepare every lunch and dinner that I eat throughout the week and pre-portion them. It is much more efficient to cook all your food in bulk than to cook each meal individually. Additionally, I try not to overcomplicate my meals. Most of the meals shown below can be prepared in under an hour or two.

The following recipes are mostly high carb/high protein recipes that I personally use to fuel my powerlifting workouts. Note that the servings sizes listed are large and you may need to cut them in half. Additionally, if your diet can't handle such a high carb load feel free to cut down on or remove the rice, potatoes, or whatever the predominant carb source is in the recipe. Likewise, if you need more fat in your diet, then feel free to cook with oil or add a side of nuts and/or seeds to a meal. If you need to add more volume to the meal, I suggest placing the meal on a bed of shredded lettuce or cabbage. The meals shown throughout this chapter are simply templates. I encourage you to modify them to meet your macronutrient and caloric needs.

## Curried Lentils Over Rice

*553 calories, 30 g protein, 106 g carbs, 1 g fat (per serving)*

Ingredients (serves 3):

- Cook 1½ cup dry green lentils (soak overnight)
- Cook ½ cup dry white rice (with a bay leaf in water)

  Curry:
- Sauté 1 medium minced onion, 2 tbsp minced ginger, 2 tbsp minced garlic
- Add 4 tsp curry powder, 1 tsp turmeric, 1 tsp cumin, 1 14-ounce can tomato puree, and a couple shakes of cayenne pepper (add more for extra spice)
- Stir the cooked lentils into the curry, simmer, and serve over the cooked rice

## Veggie Goulash

*606 calories, 34 g protein, 77 g carbs, 18 g fat (per serving)*

Ingredients (serves 5):

- 1 box protein pasta elbow macaroni
- 1 cubed eggplant (baked)
- 1 package ground beyond beef or another ground beef substitute cooked along with 8 oz. chopped white mushrooms in same pan

  Sauce:
- 2, 14-ounce cans tomato paste
- Add water to thin
- Add a few dashes of dried oregano, dried basil, garlic powder, onion powder, nutritional yeast, salt, pepper, and 2 bay leaves, then simmer
- Stir in the beyond ground beef/mushroom mix, baked cubed eggplant, and pasta into the sauce

**Protein Stir Fry**

*604 calories, 37 g protein, 69 g carbs, 20 g fat*

Ingredients (serves 1):

- ¼ block of high protein tofu, cubed and pan fried in salt, pepper, garlic powder, and ginger powder
- ½ cup of cooked edamame
- 1 cup cooked stir fry veggies
- 1 cup cooked white rice
- 1 tsp toasted sesame oil
- 1 tbsp stir fry sauce
- 2 tbsp soy sauce

**Overnight Oats**

*507 calories, 19 g protein, 65 carbs, 19 g fat*

Ingredients (serves 1):

- ½ cup oats
- ¼ cup chia seeds
- 1 cup soymilk
- 1 tbsp maple syrup
- Stir ingredients together in jar and place in fridge overnight

## Southwest Tofu Scramble over Roasted Potatoes

*451 calories, 30 g protein, 58 g carbs, 11 g fat (per serving)*

Ingredients (serves 4):

Tofu Scramble:

- Crush 2.5 packages of tofu with your hands until it looks like scrambled eggs
- Stir in lots of turmeric, paprika, onion powder, salt, chili powder, and pepper
- Add a few dashes of cumin
- Cook over medium heat in pan
- Toss in some spinach and kale to cook into the tofu scramble

Roasted Potatoes:

- Cube 8 medium red potatoes
- Put potatoes into bowl and cover in garlic powder, pepper, salt, and paprika.
- Toss chopped peppers and onion in with potatoes and bake
- Serve tofu scramble over bed of potatoes and add salsa or hot sauce if desired

## Cajun Red Beans and Rice

*544 calories, 31 g protein, 96 g carbs, 4 g fat (per serving)*

Ingredients (serves 4):

- 1 cup white rice
- 1 cup kidney beans (soaked overnight)
- Chop 4 stalks of celery, 1 one medium onion, 1 green bell pepper, and mince 2 tbsp garlic
- Add 4 cups vegetable broth to a pot with 2 bay leaves and boil kidney beans
- Add in chopped celery, onion, garlic, a dash of cayenne pepper, ½ tsp thyme, ½ tsp paprika, ½ tbsp parsley, a few dashes of Tony's creole seasoning, a dash of salt, a dash of pepper, and a splash of hot sauce.
- Simmer on low for 1 hour and 15 minutes
- Add a few drops of liquid smoke, 4 servings of sliced and fried tempeh, then simmer for 15 more minutes
- Serve over cooked rice

## Mongolian BBQ seitan

*399 calories, 44 g protein, 40 carbs, 7 g fat*

Ingredients (serves 3):

- 1 cup dry white rice
- ½ cup steamed broccoli
- 16 oz. shredded seitan fried and cooked in sauce
- For sauce, mix 2 tsp vegetable oil, ½ tsp minced ginger, 3 cloves garlic, 1/3 tsp red pepper flakes, ½ cup soy sauce, ½ cup brown sugar, 2 tsp corn starch, and 2 tbsp water
- To garnish, sprinkle chopped fresh green onion and sesame seeds

## Mini Plant-Based Fried "Chicken" Tacos

*242 calories, 11 g protein, 36 g carbs, 6 g fat*

Ingredients (serves 1):

- 2 pieces Gardein Seven Grain Crispy Tenders fried and seasoned in powdered onion, powdered garlic, chipotle seasoning, chili powder, cumin, paprika, black pepper, salt, and cayenne pepper
- 1 mini flour tortilla
- A pinch of white rice
- ½ cup of shredded cabbage or lettuce

## Nimai Delgado's Protein Buddha Bowl

*646 calories, 35 g protein, 72 g carbs, 28 g fat*

Ingredients (serves 1):

- 2 cups mixed greens salad to form a bed
- 1 medium sweet potato w/ cinnamon
- ½ cup chickpeas
- 4 oz high protein tofu cooked in Bragg liquid aminos, red pepper flakes, curry powder, garlic powder, onion powder, paprika, turmeric, and cumin
- ½ avocado
- 7 pieces broccolini
- Season entire bowl with garlic and black pepper

## Patrik Baboumian's Protein Smoothie

*720 calories, 80 g protein, 100 g carbs, 0 g fat*

Ingredients (serves 1):

- Mixed fruit
- Protein powder (Patrik uses soy isolate, pea protein isolate, or a plant-based blend)
- 1 serving glutamine
- 1 serving beta-alanine
- 5 g creatine
- 1 serving dried greens superfood powder
- Turmeric & cinnamon (for antioxidants)
- 5-10 g branched chain amino acids (BCAAs)
- Orange & mango juice

## Bradie's Monster Mass Gainer Milkshake

*1575 calories, 56 g protein, 253 g carbs, 43 g fat*

Ingredients (serves 1):

- 1 serving plant-based mass gainer protein powder
- 2 cups vanilla soymilk
- 2 cups non-dairy ice cream
- 5 tbsp chocolate syrup

# FAQ

## *What are your thoughts on the use of anabolic steroids?*

I've personally never used and at this point I don't plan to in the future, but I have no issue with those who do use. However, I think it would be a mistake to start juicing before every other variable has been optimized to the max. If you're taking roids, not training regularly, and eating like crap, you may need to reevaluate your approach.

## *Do you have any recommended training programs?*

If strength is your primary goal, I have had a lot of success with the 5/3/1 program and Westside Barbell's Conjugate Method. I am a firm believer that just about any decent program will help you make gains if implemented properly. If you're new to powerlifting, I'd recommend giving the 5/3/1 program a shot. If you're looking for a powerlifting program that's a little more advanced, then check out the Conjugate Method. There are great books out there on both programs and an endless amount of information online, so I won't waste paper by going over them here.

## *How many calories should I be eating a day?*

There are a lot of things that go into determining this and any formula you find online is just an estimate. The best way to determine how many calories you need is by trial and error. Start by tracking the average day of eating that maintains a constant body weight for you. If you want to bulk, tack on some calories to this baseline. If you want to cut, then take away calories from this baseline. After a week, weigh yourself. If you're getting the results you want, stick with this caloric intake. If nothing changes or your bodyweight went in the wrong direction, then make another small caloric adjustment for a week and repeat the process. If you are trying to cut and physically cannot reduce your calories any more than you already have, you may want to consider reverse dieting. This advanced dieting technique allows you to lose weight while eating the maximum number of calories possible. However, for this to work, you must be meticulous with calorie counting. Dr. Layne Norton has an excellent book titled *The Complete Reverse Dieting Guide* if you want to learn more about this.

## *What are your thoughts on raw vegan diets?*

I view raw vegan diets as more of a fad diet. I don't see any benefit for eating a raw vegan diet over a conventional vegan diet. Raw veganism seems way too restrictive and it is far too easy to under eat to a point where caloric intake can get dangerously low. If you're hell bent on raw veganism, I suggest tracking your calories to make sure you're eating enough and only doing the diet for a short period of time.

## *Somebody I know went on a plant-based diet and got sick. Are you sure it's safe?*

There seems to be more and more "ex-vegan" trolls popping up online who tell horror stories of health issues that they have attributed to a vegan diet. There are lots of YouTube videos of these ex-vegans telling stories of feeling sickly then eating a steak and magically feeling better. This seems to come down to nothing other than the placebo effect. It's likely all in their heads considering nutrient deficiencies can't be fixed with a single meal. It typically takes weeks to fix nutrient deficiencies, so these types of stories don't really add up. Don't get me wrong, it is possible to develop nutrient deficiencies on a vegan diet. However, it seems a lot easier to develop these same deficiencies on a standard American diet since plant-based diets tend to be more nutrient dense. Additionally, health problems pop up all the time in people. If those people are vegan around the time these health issues pop up, the diet is often falsely associated with the health issue. Overall, I think most of these people are simply suffering from the placebo effect more than anything.

## *Thoughts on plant-based pets?*

I personally don't think there is enough research out there on pet nutrition to be able to say that it is perfectly safe to put dogs and cats on an entirely plant-based diet. If you have serious ethical issues with feeding dogs and cats animal products, it is probably best to not own a pet. Hopefully, things like lab meat will be able to help solve these ethical dilemmas in the future.

## *Are you sponsored by Impossible Foods, Cronometer, or any other company?*

No.

## *Are plant-based diets safe for kids and pregnant women?*

Yes. The world's largest organization of nutritional professionals, the American Academy of Nutrition and Dietetics, has stated vegan and vegetarian diets are appropriate for all stages of the life cycle, including pregnancy, lactation, infancy, childhood, adolescence, older adulthood, and for athletes.[111]

## *I'm thinking about competing in a strength sport. How do I know when I'm ready?*

You won't ever feel truly ready. I recommend jumping into your first competition sooner rather than later. You will learn more in your first competition than you have over your entire lifting career. You're doing yourself a disservice by waiting until you're "ready."

## *Should I hire a coach if I want to compete?*

This is a difficult question and will vary person to person. If you feel confident enough to manage your diet and training or just compete casually, then you probably don't need a coach. If you're unsure how to approach training and diet or want to take things to the next level, then a coach is highly recommended. I have never used a formal coach because I enjoy being my own coach and self-teaching. When I have a training or diet question that needs answered, I turn to trusted colleagues and/or the academic literature. If you don't have these resources available to you, a coach is something that you should consider.

## *Do you do coaching?*

No.

## *How long should my training sessions be?*

This again will depend on the individual, but I'd say shoot for 45-90 min. Anything shorter than 45 minutes probably isn't enough time to perform many exercises. Any longer than 90 min and it is likely that you're wasting too much time chatting, resting, or overtraining. Additionally, after about an hour of training, maximum power output seems to drop significantly.

*I can't put on weight no matter how hard I try. What should I do?*

This is an easy one. EAT! If you're not putting on weight, there's only one thing you can do about it and that is to consume more calories. I don't want to hear that you have a freakishly fast metabolism or how you already eat so much because those are just excuses. Eat calorie dense food, eat a lot of it, and eat it often. That's all you need to do. If you're honestly incapable of eating anymore food, then I suggest consuming more liquid calories. Get some good plant-based weight gainer protein powder and blend it with some vegan ice cream, soymilk, and chocolate syrup. If you drink one of these monsters a day, are eating as much as possible, and still aren't putting on weight, then you're lying.

*How many times a week should I go to the gym?*

This will depend a lot on the induvial, their availability, and what they're training for. I can only speak from a powerlifting perspective when I say the optimum days per week for me seems to be about 4 lifts per week. This allows ample time to recover in-between intense training sessions. Back when I was training more for aesthetic than strength, I'd hit the gym about 6 days a week, but I was doing far fewer compound lifts back then and moving much less weight.

*Aren't your gains just residual strength left over from when you ate meat?*

No, not at all. I have become significantly stronger and have put on tons of muscle mass since going vegan. All this new muscle is composed entirely of proteins sourced from plants. I did not compete in powerlifting until about two years after going vegan. Sure, I played football before then, but I was not nearly as strong then as I am now as a vegan.

*Aren't all strong vegans just taking a ton of steroids?*

This is 100% false. There is a plethora of drug-tested vegan strength athletes out there, including myself. You do not need steroids to get strong on a plant-based diet. Additionally, it is not fair to say that anybody who does choose to use steroids completely owes their gains to the drug. Steroids cannot make up for poor diet and exercise habits. So, this argument that vegans would be weak without steroids is incredibly flawed.

*My performance in the gym has plateaued and I'm struggling to make gains. What should I do?*

The best way to break a plateau is to do something different. I recommend starting a new training program that is significantly different than the previous.

*Haven't humans evolved to eat meat?*

Not exactly. Sure, the human body is capable of digesting meat, but that doesn't mean it's the ideal fuel for the living machine. The idea that we should eat meat just because our ancestors did is absurd if you really think about it. Contrary to mainstream thought pushed by paleo advocates, there was no single type of diet consumed by our ancestors. They simply ate whatever they could get their hands on to survive. Even if they did consume a uniform diet of meat and vegetables, these people were lucky to live to see 30 so whatever they were doing was clearly unideal. I don't think it is worthwhile to model modern eating habits after the diet of cavemen.

# Epilogue

In a world dominated by pseudoscience, quackery, and hyperbole, I hope that I have provided some semblance of a guiding light for those interested in plant-based diets. Unfortunately, vast amounts of misinformation on nutrition have convinced people to avoid plant-based diets or to adopt them, but for the wrong reasons. I wrote this book because I recognized a void in digestible plant-based nutritional guidance for those seeking to build strength and mass. The general public is not equipped to deeply understand, nor do they have the means to access the information in academic literature on nutrition science because it is hidden behind paywalls and esoteric terminology. My goal was to offer a way to circumnavigate these boundaries with this book for those interested. I hope I have accomplished that goal.

Athletes around the world are shifting towards plant-based diets, but many of them are not the best at sharing why they are doing this with the world. It seems that many professional athletes view their plant-based diet as a trade secret to give themselves a competitive edge. Well now their secret is out. When properly planned, scientific evidence supports that a plant-based diet can provide an edge over standard omnivorous diets. A plant-based diet steers people away from junk food and toward more micronutrient dense food, increasing their intake of critical vitamins and minerals. The increased fiber intake associated with a plant-based diet improves the microbiome, further increasing micronutrient intake by promoting absorption in the gut. Faster recovery can be achieved in-between workouts by maximizing antioxidant intake and reducing the consumption of inflammatory compounds found in animal products. Blood flow can be enhanced by removing cholesterol from the diet and reducing saturated fat intake, improving exercise performance by decreasing blood viscosity and getting oxygen to the muscles more quickly. Finally, the chip on the shoulder effect will force a plant-based dieter into a beastlike mentality as they seek to prove their skeptics wrong by producing unprecedented results in the gym.

Knowledge is power and with great power, comes great responsibility. Use the knowledge provided to you in this book wisely. Understand that as soon as you publicly adopt a plant-based diet, you represent a movement. Like most members of a revolutionary movement, you will face harsh scrutiny, so you better get strong. When coupled with a well-designed exercise program, the tools provided in this book are guaranteed to make you stronger when implemented properly. However, this is all for nothing if you cannot maintain the mental strength to swim against the stream and stand up to the status quo. If you do manage to accomplish this feat, I can assure you that great rewards await you.

So, go forth. Pursue your strength goals with fervor and smash them. Prove your carnivorous brethren wrong and become stronger than them. Share your knowledge with whoever will listen. The moment when elite plant-based athletes will rise is upon us. Lead the movement by being at the forefront of it. The skeptics will slowly come around, but it will take time. Be patient. Don't reprimand the naysayers. Practice your plant-based diet with a powerful grace. Demonstrate your plant fueled strength and provide the naysayers with guidance and encouragement. Nurture them, because if you're like me, at one point you were a naysayer too. The time has come to put down this book and become part of the plant-based movement. Will you answer the call to transcend the status quo or simply remain a conformist?

# *References*

(1) Hajj, G.; Mauricio, B. M. L.; Antony, G. Is a Vegan Diet Detrimental to Endurance and Muscle Strength ? *Eur. J. Clin. Nutr.* **2020**. https://doi.org/10.1038/s41430-020-0639-y.

(2) Tomova, A.; Bukovsky, I.; Rembert, E.; Yonas, W.; Alwarith, J.; Barnard, N. D.; Kahleova, H. The Effects of Vegetarian and Vegan Diets on Gut Microbiota. *Front. Nutr.* **2019**, *6* (47). https://doi.org/10.3389/fnut.2019.00047.

(3) Noah, N. D.; Bender, A. E.; Reaidi, G. B.; Gilbert, R. J. Food Poisoning from Raw Red Kidney Beans. *Br. Med. J.* **1980**, *281* (6234), 236–237.

(4) Rodhouse, J. C.; Haugh, C. A.; Roberts, D.; Gilbert, R. J. Red Kidney Bean Poisoning in the UK: An Analysis of 50 Suspected Incidents between 1976 and 1989. *Epidemiol. Infect.* **1990**, *105* (3), 485–491. https://doi.org/10.1017/S095026880004810X.

(5) Quagliani, D.; Felt-Gunderson, P. Closing America's Fiber Intake Gap: Communication Strategies From a Food and Fiber Summit. *Am. J. Lifestyle Med.* **2017**, *11* (1), 80–85. https://doi.org/10.1177/1559827615588079.

(6) Anderson, J. W.; Baird, P.; Davis, R. H.; Ferreri, S.; Knudtson, M.; Koraym, A.; Waters, V.; Williams, C. L. Health Benefits of Dietary Fiber. *Nutr. Rev.* **2009**, *67* (4), 188–205. https://doi.org/10.1111/j.1753-4887.2009.00189.x.

(7) Beavers, K. M.; Brinkley, T. E.; Nicklas, B. J. Effect of Exercise Training on Chronic Inflammation. *Clin. Chim. Acta* **2010**, *411* (11–12), 785–793. https://doi.org/10.1016/j.cca.2010.02.069.

(8) Baker, M. E.; DeCesare, K. N.; Johnson, A.; Kress, K. S.; Inman, C. L.; Weiss, E. P. Short-Term Mediterranean Diet Improves Endurance Exercise Performance: A Randomized-Sequence Crossover Trial. *J. Am. Coll. Nutr.* **2019**, *38* (7), 597–605. https://doi.org/10.1080/07315724.2019.1568322.

(9) Sun, X.; Jiao, X.; Ma, Y.; Liu, Y.; Zhang, L.; He, Y.; Chen, Y. Trimethylamine N-Oxide Induces Inflammation and Endothelial Dysfunction in Human Umbilical Vein Endothelial Cells via Activating ROS-TXNIP-NLRP3 Inflammasome. *Biochem. Biophys. Res. Commun.* **2016**, *481* (1–2), 63–70. https://doi.org/10.1016/j.bbrc.2016.11.017.

(10) Li, Z.; Wong, A.; Henning, S. M.; Zhang, Y.; Jones, A.; Zerlin, A.; Thames, G.; Bowerman, S.; Tseng, C. H.; Heber, D. Hass Avocado Modulates Postprandial Vascular Reactivity and Postprandial Inflammatory Responses to a Hamburger Meal in Healthy Volunteers. *Food Funct.* **2013**, *4* (3), 384–391. https://doi.org/10.1039/c2fo30226h.

(11) Wessling-Resnick, M. Iron Homeostasis and the Inflammatory Response. *Annu. Rev. Nutr.* **2010**, *30* (1), 105–122. https://doi.org/10.1146/annurev.nutr.012809.104804.

(12) World Health Organization International Agency for Research on Cancer. IARC Monographs Evaluate Consumption of Red Meat and Processed Meat and Cancer Risk. 26 October **2015**, 1–2. Press release. www.who.int/features/qa/cancer-red-meat/en/.

(13) Robblee, M. M.; Kim, C. C.; Abate, J. P.; Valdearcos, M.; Sandlund, K. L. M.; Shenoy, M. K.; Volmer, R.; Iwawaki, T.; Koliwad, S. K. Saturated Fatty Acids Engage an IRE1α-Dependent Pathway to Activate the NLRP3 Inflammasome in Myeloid Cells. *Cell Rep.* **2016**, *14* (11), 2611–2623. https://doi.org/10.1016/j.celrep.2016.02.053.

(14) Key, T. J.; Appleby, P. N.; Rosell, M. S. Health Effects of Vegetarian and Vegan Diets. *Proc. Nutr. Soc.* **2006**, *65* (1), 35–41. https://doi.org/10.1079/pns2005481.

(15) Carlsen, M. H.; Halvorsen, B. L.; Holte, K.; Bøhn, S. K.; Dragland, S.; Sampson, L.; Willey, C.; Senoo, H.; Umezono, Y.; Sanada, C.; et al. The Total Antioxidant Content of More than 3100 Foods, Beverages, Spices, Herbs and Supplements Used Worldwide. *Nutr. J.* **2010**, *9* (1), 1–11. https://doi.org/10.1186/1475-2891-9-3.

(16) Sutliffe, J. T.; Wilson, L. D.; de Heer, H. D.; Foster, R. L.; Carnot, M. J. C-Reactive Protein Response to a Vegan Lifestyle Intervention. *Complement. Ther. Med.* **2015**, *23* (1), 32–37. https://doi.org/10.1016/j.ctim.2014.11.001.

(17) Hutchison, A. T.; Flieller, E. B.; Dillon, K. J.; Leverett, B. D. Black Currant Nectar Reduces Muscle Damage and Inflammation Following a Bout of High-Intensity Eccentric Contractions. *J. Diet. Suppl.* **2016**, *13* (1), 1–15. https://doi.org/10.3109/19390211.2014.952864.

(18) Howatson, G.; McHugh, M. P.; Hill, J. A.; Brouner, J.; Jewell, A. P.; Van Someren, K. A.; Shave, R. E.; Howatson, S. A. Influence of Tart Cherry Juice on Indices of Recovery Following Marathon Running. *Scand. J. Med. Sci. Sport.* **2010**, *20* (6), 843–852. https://doi.org/10.1111/j.1600-0838.2009.01005.x.

(19) Bowtell, J. L.; Sumners, D. P.; Dyer, A.; Fox, P.; Mileva, K. N. Montmorency Cherry Juice Reduces Muscle Damage Caused by Intensive Strength Exercise. *Med. Sci. Sports Exerc.* **2011**, *43* (8), 1544–1551. https://doi.org/10.1249/MSS.0b013e31820e5adc.

(20) Trombold, J. R.; Reinfeld, A. S.; Casler, J. R.; Coyle, E. F. The Effect of Pomegranate Juice Supplementation on Strength and Soreness after Eccentric Exercise. *J. Strength Cond. Res.* **2011**, *25* (7), 1782–1788. https://doi.org/10.1519/JSC.0b013e318220d992.

(21) Tarazona-Díaz, M. P.; Alacid, F.; Carrasco, M.; Martínez, I.; Aguayo, E. Watermelon Juice: Potential Functional Drink for Sore Muscle Relief in Athletes. *J. Agric. Food Chem.* **2013**, *61* (31), 7522–7528. https://doi.org/10.1021/jf400964r.

(22) Barnard, N. D.; Goldman, D. M.; Loomis, J. F.; Kahleova, H.; Levin, S. M.; Neabore, S.; Batts, T. C. Plant-Based Diets for Cardiovascular Safety and Performance in Endurance Sports. *Nutrients* **2019**, *11* (1), 1–10. https://doi.org/10.3390/nu11010130.

(23) McCarty, M. F. Favorable Impact of a Vegan Diet with Exercise on Hemorheology: Implications for Control of Diabetic Neuropathy. *Med. Hypotheses* **2002**, *58* (6), 476–486. https://doi.org/10.1054/mehy.2001.1456.

(24) Ernst, E.; Pietsch, L.; Matrai, A.; Eisenberg, J. Blood Rheology in Vegetarians. *Br. J. Nutr.* **1986**, *56* (3), 555–560. https://doi.org/10.1079/bjn19860136.

(25) El-Sayed, M. S.; Ali, N.; Ali, Z. E. S. Haemorheology in Exercise and Training. *Sport. Med.* **2005**, *35* (8), 649–670. https://doi.org/10.2165/00007256-200535080-00001.

(26) Smith, M. M.; Lucas, A. R.; Hamlin, R. L.; Devor, S. T. Associations among Hemorheological Factors and Maximal Oxygen Consumption. Is There a Role for Blood Viscosity in Explaining Athletic Performance? *Clin. Hemorheol. Microcirc.* **2015**, *60* (4), 347–362. https://doi.org/10.3233/CH-131708.

(27) Heron, M. National Vital Statistics Reports Deaths: Leading Causes for 2013. *Natl. vital Stat. reports from Centers Dis. Control Prev. Natl. Cent. Heal. Stat. Natl. Vital Stat. Syst.* **2016**, *65* (2), 1–95.

(28) Kim, H.; Caulfield, L. E.; Garcia-Larsen, V.; Steffen, L. M.; Coresh, J.; Rebholz, C. M. Plant-Based Diets Are Associated With a Lower Risk of Incident Cardiovascular Disease, Cardiovascular Disease Mortality, and All-Cause Mortality in a General Population of Middle-Aged Adults. *J. Am. Heart Assoc.* **2019**, *8* (16). https://doi.org/10.1161/JAHA.119.012865.

(29) Yamada, T.; Hara, K.; Umematsu, H.; Suzuki, R.; Kadowaki, T. Erectile Dysfunction and Cardiovascular Events in Diabetic Men: A Meta-Analysis of Observational Studies. *PLoS One* **2012**, *7* (9). https://doi.org/10.1371/journal.pone.0043673.

(30) Schwartz, B. G.; Kloner, R. A. Cardiovascular Implications of Erectile Dysfunction. *Circulation* **2011**, *123* (21), 609–611. https://doi.org/10.1161/CIRCULATIONAHA.110.017681.

(31) Wang, F.; Dai, S.; Wang, M.; Morrison, H. Erectile Dysfunction and Fruit/Vegetable Consumption among Diabetic Canadian Men. *Urology* **2013**, *82* (6), 1330–1335. https://doi.org/10.1016/j.urology.2013.07.061.

(32) Cassidy, A.; Franz, M.; Rimm, E. B. Dietary Flavonoid Intake and Incidence of Erectile Dysfunction. *Am. J. Clin. Nutr.* **2016**, *103* (2), 534–541. https://doi.org/10.3945/ajcn.115.122010.

(33) Phillips, S. M.; van Loon, L. J. C. Dietary Protein for Athletes: From Requirements to Optimum Adaptation. *J. Sports Sci.* **2011**, *29* (S1). https://doi.org/10.1080/02640414.2011.619204.

(34) Gorissen, S. H.; Horstman, A. M.; Franssen, R.; Crombag, J. J.; Langer, H.; Bierau, J.; Respondek, F.; van Loon, L. J. Ingestion of Wheat Protein Increases In Vivo Muscle Protein Synthesis Rates in Healthy Older Men in a Randomized Trial. *J. Nutr.* **2016**, *146* (9), 1651–1659. https://doi.org/10.3945/jn.116.231340.

(35) Young, V. R.; Pellett, P. L. Plant Proteins in Relation to Human Protein and Amino Acid Nutrition. *Am. J. Clin. Nutr.* **1994**, *59* (5 Suppl.). https://doi.org/10.1093/ajcn/59.5.1203S.

(36) Schoenfeld, B. J.; Aragon, A. A. How Much Protein Can the Body Use in a Single Meal for Muscle-Building? Implications for Daily Protein Distribution. *J. Int. Soc. Sports Nutr.* **2018**, *15* (10), 4–9.

(37) Reidy, P. T.; Rasmussen, B. B. Role of Ingested Amino Acids and Protein in the Promotion of Resistance Exercise–Induced Muscle Protein Anabolism. *J. Nutr.* **2016**, *146* (2), 155–183. https://doi.org/10.3945/jn.114.203208.

(38) Martinez, J.; Lewi, J. An Unusual Case of Gynecomastia Associated with Soy Product Consumption. *Endocr. Pract.* **2008**, *14* (4), 415–418. https://doi.org/10.4158/EP.14.4.415.

(39) Nagata, C.; Takatsuka, N.; Shimizu, H.; Hayashi, H.; Akamatsu, T.; Murase, K. Effect of Soymilk Consumption on Serum Estrogen and Androgen Concentrations in Japanese Men. *Cancer Epidemiol. Biomarkers Prev.* **2001**, *10* (3), 179–184.

(40) Kalman, D.; Feldman, S.; Martinez, M.; Krieger, D. R.; Tallon, M. J. Effect of Protein Source and Resistance Training on Body Composition and Sex Hormones. *J. Int. Soc. Sports Nutr.* **2007**, *4* (1), 4. https://doi.org/10.1186/1550-2783-4-4.

(41) Maskarinec, G.; Morimoto, Y.; Hebshi, S.; Sharma, S.; Franke, A. A.; Stanczyk, F. Z. Serum Prostate-Specific Antigen but Not Testosterone Levels Decrease in a Randomized Soy Intervention among Men. *Eur. J. Clin. Nutr.* **2006**, *60* (12), 1423–1429. https://doi.org/10.1038/sj.ejcn.1602473.

(42) Deibert, P.; Solleder, F.; König, D.; Vitolins, M. Z.; Dickhuth, H. H.; Gollhofer, A.; Berg, A. Soy Protein Based Supplementation Supports Metabolic Effects of Resistance Training in Previously Untrained Middle Aged Males. *Aging Male* **2011**, *14* (4), 273–279. https://doi.org/10.3109/13685538.2011.565091.

(43) Hamilton-Reeves, J. M.; Vazquez, G.; Duval, S. J.; Phipps, W. R.; Kurzer, M. S.; Messina, M. J. Clinical Studies Show No Effects of Soy Protein or Isoflavones on Reproductive Hormones in Men: Results of a Meta-Analysis. *Fertil. Steril.* **2010**, *94* (3), 997–1007. https://doi.org/10.1016/j.fertnstert.2009.04.038.

(44) Pan, L.; Xia, X.; Feng, Y.; Jiang, C.; Cui, Y.; Huang, Y. Exposure of Juvenile Rats to the Phytoestrogen Daidzein Impairs Erectile Function in a Dose-Related Manner in Adulthood. *J. Androl.* **2008**, *29* (1), 55–62. https://doi.org/10.2164/jandrol.107.003392.

(45) Messina, M. Soybean Isoflavone Exposure Does Not Have Feminizing Effects on Men: A Critical Examination of the Clinical Evidence. *Fertil. Steril.* **2010**, *93* (7), 2095–2104. https://doi.org/10.1016/j.fertnstert.2010.03.002.

(46) Malekinejad, H.; Rezabakhsh, A. Hormones in Dairy Foods and Their Impact on Public Health- A Narrative Review Article. *Iran. J. Public Health* **2015**, *44* (6), 742–758.

(47) Joy, J. M.; Lowery, R. P.; Wilson, J. M.; Purpura, M.; De Souza, E. O.; Wilson, S. M.; Kalman, D. S.; Dudeck, J. E.; Jäger, R. The Effects of 8 Weeks of Whey or Rice Protein Supplementation on Body Composition and Exercise Performance. *Nutr. J.* **2013**, *12* (1), 1–7. https://doi.org/10.1186/1475-2891-12-86.

(48) Banaszek, A.; Townsend, J. R.; Bender, D.; Vantrease, W. C.; Marshall, A. C.; Johnson, K. D. The Effects of Whey vs. Pea Protein on Physical Adaptations Following 8-Weeks of High-Intensity Functional Training (HIFT): A Pilot Study. *Sports* **2019**, *7* (1), 12. https://doi.org/10.3390/sports7010012.

(49) Minevich, J.; Olson, M. A.; Mannion, J. P.; Boublik, J. H.; McPherson, J. O.; Lowery, R. P.; Shields, K.; Sharp, M.; De Souza, E. O.; Wilson, J. M.; et al. Digestive Enzymes Reduce Quality Differences between Plant and Animal Proteins: A Double-Blind Crossover Study. *J. Int. Soc. Sports Nutr.* **2015**, *12* (S1), 9–10. https://doi.org/10.1186/1550-2783-12-s1-p26.

(50) Gardner, C. D.; Trepanowski, J. F.; Gobbo, L. C. D.; Hauser, M. E.; Rigdon, J.; Ioannidis, J. P. A.; Desai, M.; King, A. C. Effect of Low-Fat VS Low-Carbohydrate Diet on 12-Month Weight Loss in Overweight Adults and the Association with Genotype Pattern or Insulin Secretion: the DIETFITS Randomized Clinical Trial. *JAMA - J. Am. Med. Assoc.* **2018**, *319* (7), 667–679. https://doi.org/10.1001/jama.2018.0245.

(51) Hall, K. D.; Guo, J.; Courville, A. B.; Boring, J.; Brychta, R.; Kong, Y.; Darcey, V.; Forde, C. G.; Gharib, A. M.; Gallagher, I.; et al. A Plant-Based, Low-Fat Diet Decreases Ad Libitum Energy Intake Compared to an Animal-Based, Ketogenic Diet: An Inpatient Randomized Controlled Trial. 6 May **2020**. Preprint. https://doi.org/10.31232/osf.io/rdjfb

(52) Thomas, D. T.; Burke, L. M.; Erdman, K. A. Nutrition and Athletic Performance. *Med. Sci. Sports Exerc.* **2016**, *48* (3), 543–568. https://doi.org/10.1249/MSS.0000000000000852.

(53) Butki, B. D.; Baumstark, J.; Driver, S. Effects of a Carbohydrate-Restricted Diet on Affective Responses to Acute Exercise among Physically Active Participants. *Percept. Mot. Skills* **2003**, *96* (2), 607–615. https://doi.org/10.2466/pms.2003.96.2.607.

(54) White, A. M.; Johnston, C. S.; Swan, P. D.; Tjonn, S. L.; Sears, B. Blood Ketones Are Directly Related to Fatigue and Perceived Effort during Exercise in Overweight Adults Adhering to Low-Carbohydrate Diets for Weight Loss: A Pilot Study. *J. Am. Diet. Assoc.* **2007**, *107* (10), 1792–1796. https://doi.org/10.1016/j.jada.2007.07.009.

(55) Keith, R. E.; O'Keeffe, K. A.; Blessing, D. L.; Wilson, G. D. Alterations in Dietary Carbohydrate, Protein, and Fat Intake and Mood State in Trained Female Cyclists. *Medicine and Science in Sports and Exercise.* **1991**, 23 (2), 212–216. https://doi.org/10.1249/00005768-199102000-00011.

(56) Panel on Macronutrients, Panel on the Definition of Dietary Fiber, Subcommittee on Upper Reference Levels of Nutrients, Subcommittee on Interpretation and Uses of Dietary Reference Intakes, and the Standing Committee on the Scientific Evaluation of Dietary Reference Intakes. *Dietary Reference Intakes for Energy, Carbohydrate, Fiber, Fat, Fatty Acids, Cholesterol, Protein, and Amino Acids*. Institute of Medicince of the National Academies. **2005**.

(57) Holt, S. H. A.; Brand Miller, J. C.; Petocz, P.; Farmakalidis, E. A Satiety Index of Common Foods. *Eur. J. Clin. Nutr.* **1995**, *49* (9), 675–690.

(58) LeBlanc, J. G.; Milani, C.; de Giori, G. S.; Sesma, F.; van Sinderen, D.; Ventura, M. Bacteria as Vitamin Suppliers to Their Host: A Gut Microbiota Perspective. *Curr. Opin. Biotechnol.* **2013**, *24* (2), 160–168. https://doi.org/10.1016/j.copbio.2012.08.005.

(59) Tucker, K. L.; Rich, S.; Rosenberg, I.; Jacques, P.; Dallal, G.; Wilson, P. W. F.; Selhub, J. Plasma Vitamin B-12 Concentrations Relate to Intake Source in the Framingham Offspring Study. *Am. J. Clin. Nutr.* **2000**, *71* (2), 514–522. https://doi.org/10.1093/ajcn/71.2.514.

(60) Branch, J. D. Effect of Creatine Supplementation on Body Composition and Performance: A Meta-Analysis. *Int. J. Sport Nutr. Exerc. Metab.* **2003**, *13* (2), 198–226. https://doi.org/10.1123/ijsnem.13.2.198.

(61) Butts, J.; Jacobs, B.; Silvis, M. Creatine Use in Sports. *Sports Health* **2018**, *10* (1), 31–34. https://doi.org/10.1177/1941738117737248.

(62) Hultman, E.; Söderlund, K.; Timmons, J. A.; Cederblad, G.; Greenhaff, P. L. Muscle Creatine Loading in Men. *J. Appl. Physiol.* **1996**, *81* (1), 232–237. https://doi.org/10.1152/jappl.1996.81.1.232.

(63) Pittas, G.; Hazell, M. D.; Simpson, E. J.; Greenhaff, P. L. Optimization of Insulin-Mediated Creatine Retention during Creatine Feeding in Humans. *J. Sports Sci.* **2010**, *28* (1), 67–74. https://doi.org/10.1080/02640410903390071.

(64) Ostojic, S. M.; Ahmetovic, Z. Gastrointestinal Distress after Creatine Supplementation in Athletes: Are Side Effects Dose Dependent? *Res. Sport. Med.* **2008**, *16* (1), 15–22. https://doi.org/10.1080/15438620701693280.

(65) Cummings, J. H.; MacFarlane, G. T. Role of Intestinal Bacteria in Nutrient Metabolism. *Clin. Nutr.* **1997**, *16* (1), 3–11. https://doi.org/10.1016/S0261-5614(97)80252-X.

(66) Shen, J.; Obin, M. S.; Zhao, L. The Gut Microbiota, Obesity and Insulin Resistance. *Mol. Aspects Med.* **2013**, *34* (1), 39–58. https://doi.org/10.1016/j.mam.2012.11.001.

(67) Norris, V.; Molina, F.; Gewirtzc, A. T. Hypothesis: Bacteria Control Host Appetites. *J. Bacteriol.* **2013**, *195* (3), 411–416. https://doi.org/10.1128/JB.01384-12.

(68) Forrest, K. Y. Z.; Stuhldreher, W. L. Prevalence and Correlates of Vitamin D Deficiency in US Adults. *Nutr. Res.* **2011**, *31* (1), 48–54. https://doi.org/10.1016/j.nutres.2010.12.001.

(69) Ross, C. A.; Taylor C. L.; Yaktine A. L.; Heather B. DV. *Dietary Reference Intakes for Vitamin D and Calcium*; Institute of Medicince of the National Academies. **2011**. https://doi.org/10.1016/j.crma.2018.11.003.

(70) Riazi, R.; Wykes, L. J.; Ball, R. O.; Pencharz, P. B. The Total Branched-Chain Amino Acid Requirement in Young Healthy Adult Men Determined by Indicator Amino Acid Oxidation by Use of l-[1-13C]Phenylalanine. *J. Nutr.* **2003**, *133* (5), 1383–1389. https://doi.org/10.1093/jn/133.5.1383.

(71) Kimball, S. R.; Jefferson, L. S. Signaling Pathways and Molecular Mechanisms through Which Branched-Chain Amino Acids Mediate Translational Control of Protein Synthesis. *J. Nutr.* **2006**, *136* (1), 227S-231S. https://doi.org/10.1093/jn/136.1.227s.

(72) Blomstrand, E.; Hassmén, P.; Ek, S.; Ekblom, B.; Newsholme, E. A. Influence of Ingesting a Solution of Branched-Chain Amino Acids on Perceived Exertion during Exercise. *Acta Physiol. Scand.* **1997**, *159* (1), 41–49. https://doi.org/10.1046/j.1365-201X.1997.547327000.x.

(73) Howatson, G.; Hoad, M.; Goodall, S.; Tallent, J.; Bell, P. G.; French, D. N. Exercise-Induced Muscle Damage Is Reduced in Resistance-Trained Males by Branched Chain Amino Acids: A Randomized, Double-Blind, Placebo Controlled Study. *J. Int. Soc. Sports Nutr.* **2012**, *20* (9), 1–7. https://doi.org/10.3177/jnsv.46.71.

(74) Shimomura, Y.; Shimomura, Y.; Inaguma, A.; Watanabe, S.; Yamamoto, Y.; Muramatsu, Y.; Bajotto, G.; Sato, J.; Shimomura, N.; Kobayashi, H.; et al. Branched-Chain Amino Acid Supplementation Before Squat Exercise and Delayed-Onset Muscle Soreness. *Int. J. Sport Nutr. Exerc. Metab.* **2010**, *20*, 236–244.

(75) Leahy, D. T.; Pintauro, S. J. Branched-Chain Amino Acid Plus Glucose Supplement Reduces Exercise-Induced Delayed Onset Muscle Soreness in College-Age Females. *ISRN Nutr.* **2013**, *2013*, 1–5. https://doi.org/10.5402/2013/921972.

(76) Wandrag, L.; Brett, S. J.; Frost, G.; Hickson, M. Impact of Supplementation with Amino Acids or Their Metabolites on Muscle Wasting in Patients with Critical Illness or Other Muscle Wasting Illness: A Systematic Review. *J. Hum. Nutr. Diet.* **2015**, *28* (4), 313–330. https://doi.org/10.1111/jhn.12238.

(77) Grosso, G.; Galvano, F.; Marventano, S.; Malaguarnera, M.; Bucolo, C.; Drago, F.; Caraci, F. Omega-3 Fatty Acids and Depression: Scientific Evidence and Biological Mechanisms. *Oxid. Med. Cell. Longev.* **2014**. https://doi.org/10.1155/2014/313570.

(78) Kruger, M. C.; Horrobin, D. F. Calcium Metabolism, Osteoporosis and Essential Fatty Acids: A Review. *Prog. Lipid Res.* **1997**, *36* (2–3), 131–151. https://doi.org/10.1016/S0163-7827(97)00007-6.

(79) Morel, F. M. M.; Kraepiel, A. M. L.; Amyot, M. The Chemical Cycle and Bioaccumulation of Mercury. *Annu. Rev. Ecol. Syst.* **1998**, *29*, 543–566. https://doi.org/10.1146/annurev.ecolsys.29.1.543.

(80) Saper, R. B.; Rash, R. Zinc: An Essential Micronutrient. *Am. Fam. Physician* **2009**, *79* (9), 768–772.

(81) Hemilä, H. Zinc Lozenges and the Common Cold: A Meta-Analysis Comparing Zinc Acetate and Zinc Gluconate, and the Role of Zinc Dosage. *JRSM Open* **2017**, *8* (5), 205427041769429. https://doi.org/10.1177/2054270417694291.

(82) Ranasinghe, P.; Wathurapatha, W. S.; Ishara, M. H.; Jayawardana, R.; Galappatthy, P.; Katulanda, P.; Constantine, G. R. Effects of Zinc Supplementation on Serum Lipids: A Systematic Review and Meta-Analysis. *Nutr. Metab.* **2015**, *12* (1). https://doi.org/10.1186/s12986-015-0023-4.

(83) Prasad, A. S.; Bao, B.; Beck, F. W. J.; Kucuk, O.; Sarkar, F. H. Antioxidant Effect of Zinc in Humans. *Free Radic. Biol. Med.* **2004**, *37* (8), 1182–1190. https://doi.org/10.1016/j.freeradbiomed.2004.07.007.

(84) Foster, M.; Chu, A.; Petocz, P.; Samman, S. Effect of Vegetarian Diets on Zinc Status: A Systematic Review and Meta-Analysis of Studies in Humans. *J. Sci. Food Agric.* **2013**, *93* (10), 2362–2371. https://doi.org/10.1002/jsfa.6179.

(85) Alekseeva, L. I.; Sharapova, E. P.; Kashevarova, N. G.; Taskina, E. A.; Anikin, S. G.; Korotkova, T. A.; Pyanykh, S. E. Use of ARTRA MSM FORTE in Patients with Knee Osteoarthritis: Results of a Randomized Openlabel Comparative Study of the Efficacy and Tolerability of the Drug. *Ter. Arkh.* **2015**, *87* (12), 49–54. https://doi.org/10.17116/terarkh2015871249-54.

(86) Lubis, A. M. T.; Siagian, C.; Wonggokusuma, E.; Marsetyo, A. F.; Setyohadi, B. Comparison of Glucosamine-Chondroitin Sulfate with and without Methylsulfonylmethane in Grade I-II Knee Osteoarthritis: A Double Blind Randomized Controlled Trial. *Acta Med. Indones.* **2017**, *49* (2), 105–111.

(87) Wandel, S.; Jüni, P.; Tendal, B.; Nüesch, E.; Villiger, P. M.; Welton, N. J.; Reichenbach, S.; Trelle, S. Effects of Glucosamine, Chondroitin, or Placebo in Patients with Osteoarthritis of Hip or Knee: Network Meta-Analysis. *BMJ* **2010**, *341* (7775), 711. https://doi.org/10.1136/bmj.c4675.

(88) Kantor, E. D.; Lampe, J. W.; Navarro, S. L.; Song, X.; Milne, G. L.; White, E. Associations between Glucosamine and Chondroitin Supplement Use and Biomarkers of Systemic Inflammation. *J. Altern. Complement. Med.* **2014**, *20* (6), 479–485. https://doi.org/10.1089/acm.2013.0323.

(89) Momomura, R.; Naito, K.; Igarashi, M.; Watari, T.; Terakado, A.; Oike, S.; Sakamoto, K.; Nagaoka, I.; Kaneko, K. Evaluation of the Effect of Glucosamine Administration on Biomarkers of Cartilage and Bone Metabolism in Bicycle Racers. *Mol. Med. Rep.* **2013**, *7* (3), 742–746. https://doi.org/10.3892/mmr.2013.1289.

(90) Rosanoff, A.; Weaver, C. M.; Rude, R. K. Suboptimal Magnesium Status in the United States: Are the Health Consequences Underestimated? *Nutr. Rev.* **2012**, *70* (3), 153–164. https://doi.org/10.1111/j.1753-4887.2011.00465.x.

(91) Zhang, Y.; Xun, P.; Wang, R.; Mao, L.; He, K. Can Magnesium Enhance Exercise Performance? *Nutrients* **2017**, *9* (9), 1–10. https://doi.org/10.3390/nu9090946.

(92) Derave, W.; Özdemir, M. S.; Harris, R. C.; Pottier, A.; Reyngoudt, H.; Koppo, K.; Wise, J. A.; Achten, E. β-Alanine Supplementation Augments Muscle Carnosine Content and Attenuates Fatigue during Repeated Isokinetic Contraction Bouts in Trained Sprinters. *J. Appl. Physiol.* **2007**, *103* (5), 1736–1743. https://doi.org/10.1152/japplphysiol.00397.2007.

(93) Everaert, I.; Stegen, S.; Vanheel, B.; Taes, Y.; Derave, W. Effect of Beta-Alanine and Carnosine Supplementation on Muscle Contractility in Mice. *Med. Sci. Sports Exerc.* **2013**, *45* (1), 43–51. https://doi.org/10.1249/MSS.0b013e31826cdb68.

(94) Trexler, E. T.; Smith-Ryan, A. E.; Stout, J. R.; Hoffman, J. R.; Wilborn, C. D.; Sale, C.; Kreider, R. B.; Jäger, R.; Earnest, C. P.; Bannock, L.; et al. International Society of Sports Nutrition Position Stand: Beta-Alanine. *J. Int. Soc. Sports Nutr.* **2015**, *12* (1), 1–14. https://doi.org/10.1186/s12970-015-0090-y.

(95) Stellingwerff, T.; Anwander, H.; Egger, A.; Buehler, T.; Kreis, R.; Decombaz, J.; Boesch, C. Effect of Two β-Alanine Dosing Protocols on Muscle Carnosine Synthesis and Washout. *Amino Acids* **2012**, *42* (6), 2461–2472. https://doi.org/10.1007/s00726-011-1054-4.

(96) Churchward-Venne, T. A.; Burd, N. A.; Mitchell, C. J.; West, D. W. D.; Philp, A.; Marcotte, G. R.; Baker, S. K.; Baar, K.; Phillips, S. M. Supplementation of a Suboptimal Protein Dose with Leucine or Essential Amino Acids: Effects on Myofibrillar Protein Synthesis at Rest and Following Resistance Exercise in Men. *J. Physiol.* **2012**, *590* (11), 2751–2765. https://doi.org/10.1113/jphysiol.2012.228833.

(97) Murphy, C. H.; Saddler, N. I.; Devries, M. C.; McGlory, C.; Baker, S. K.; Phillips, S. M. Leucine Supplementation Enhances Integrative Myofibrillar Protein Synthesis in Free-Living Older Men Consuming Lower-and Higher-Protein Diets: A Parallel-Group Crossover Study1. *Am. J. Clin. Nutr.* **2016**, *104* (6), 1594–1606. https://doi.org/10.3945/ajcn.116.136424.

(98) Gorissen, S. H. M.; Burd, N. A.; Hamer, H. M.; Gijsen, A. P.; Groen, B. B.; Van Loon, L. J. C. Carbohydrate Coingestion Delays Dietary Protein Digestion and Absorption but Does Not Modulate Postprandial Muscle Protein Accretion. *J. Clin. Endocrinol. Metab.* **2014**, *99* (6), 2250–2258. https://doi.org/10.1210/jc.2013-3970.

(99) Craig, W. J.; Mangels, A. R. Position of the American Dietetic Association: Vegetarian Diets. *J. Am. Diet. Assoc.* **2009**, *109* (7), 1266–1282. https://doi.org/10.1016/j.jada.2009.05.027.

(100) Davey, G. K.; Spencer, E. A.; Appleby, P. N.; Allen, N. E.; Knox, K. H.; Key, T. J. EPIC–Oxford:Lifestyle Characteristics and Nutrient Intakes in a Cohort of 33 883 Meat-Eaters and 31 546 Non Meat-Eaters in the UK. *Public Health Nutr.* **2003**, *6* (3), 259–268. https://doi.org/10.1079/phn2002430.

(101) Hunt, J. R. Bioavailability of Iron, Zinc, and Other Trace Minerals from Vegetarian Diets. *Am. J. Clin. Nutr.* **2003**, *78* (3 Suppl.). https://doi.org/10.1093/ajcn/78.3.633s.

(102) Intakes, D. R.; Vanadium, U.; Levels, Z. R.; Intakes, D. R.; Committee, S.; Evaluation, S.; Reference, D.; Isbn, I.; Pdf, T.; Press, N. A.; et al. *Dietary Reference Intakes for Vitamin A, Vitamin K, Arsenic, Boron, Chromium, Copper, Iodine, Iron, Manganese, Molybdenum, Nickel, Silicon, Vanadium, and* Zinc. National Academy of Science Institute of Medicine. **2002**.

(103) Le, C. H. H. The Prevalence of Anemia and Moderate-Severe Anemia in the US Population (NHANES 2003-2012). *PLoS One* **2016**, *11* (11), 1–14. https://doi.org/10.1371/journal.pone.0166635.

(104) Hallberg, L.; Hulthén, L. Prediction of Dietary Iron Absorption: An Algorithm for Calculating Absorption and Bioavailability of Dietary Iron. *Am. J. Clin. Nutr.* **2000**, *71* (5), 1147–1160. https://doi.org/10.1093/ajcn/71.5.1147.

(105) Ziegler, E. E. Consumption of Cow's Milk as a Cause of Iron Deficiency in Infants and Toddlers. *Nutr. Rev.* **2011**, *69* (Suppl. 1), 37–42. https://doi.org/10.1111/j.1753-4887.2011.00431.x.

(106) Mangels, A. R. Bone Nutrients for Vegetarians. *Am. J. Clin. Nutr.* **2014**, *100*, 469S-475S. https://doi.org/10.3945/ajcn.113.071423.2.

(107) Iguacel, I.; Miguel-Berges, M. L.; Gómez-Bruton, A.; Moreno, L. A.; Julián, C. Veganism, Vegetarianism, Bone Mineral Density, and Fracture Risk: A Systematic Review and Meta-Analysis. *Nutr. Rev.* **2019**, *77* (1), 1–18. https://doi.org/10.1093/nutrit/nuy045.

(108) Appleby, P.; Roddam, A.; Allen, N.; Key, T. Comparative Fracture Risk in Vegetarians and Nonvegetarians in EPIC-Oxford. *Eur. J. Clin. Nutr.* **2007**, *61* (12), 1400–1406. https://doi.org/10.1038/sj.ejcn.1602659.

(109) Kita, P. The Mountain Says He's Open to Giving a Vegan Diet a Try. *Men's Health*. 28 October **2019**. https://www.menshealth.com/nutrition/a29613285/the-mountain-vegan-diet/

(110) Patrik Baboumian. WHAT I EAT IN A DAY / VEGAN STRONGMAN. *YouTube*. 15 July **2019**. https://www.youtube.com/watch?v=aPJWOWePRGs

(111) Melina, V.; Craig, W.; Levin, S. Position of the Academy of Nutrition and Dietetics: Vegetarian Diets. *J. Acad. Nutr. Diet.* **2016**, *116* (12), 1970–1980. https://doi.org/10.1016/j.jand.2016.09.025.

# Other Published Works by Bradie S. Crandall

Preparing for the Worst: The Case for Solar Geoengineering Research and Oversight. *Journal of Engineering & Public Policy.* **2019**.

Desulfurization of Liquid Hydrocarbon Fuels with Microporous and Mesoporous Materials: Metal-Organic Frameworks, Zeolites, and Mesoporous Silicas. *Industrial & Engineering Chemistry Research.* **2019**.

Activity and stability of NiCe@SiO$_2$ multi–yolk–shell nanotube catalyst for tri-reforming of methane. *Applied Catalysis B: Environmental.* **2019.**

Printed in Great Britain
by Amazon